RAISING CATS NATURALLY

*How to care for your cat
the way nature intended*

By Michelle T. Bernard

Raising Cats Naturally

How to care for your cat

the way nature intended

Michelle T. Bernard

Published by:
    Blakkatz Publishing
    Lincolnton, NC 28092, U.S.A.
    mbernard@blakkatz.com
    http://www.blakkatz.com

RAISING CATS NATURALLY
How to care for your cat the way nature intended
Copyright 2003© Michelle T. Bernard

All rights reserved. No part of this book may be reproduced or transmitted in any form or by any means, electronic or mechanical, including photocopying, recording or by any information storage and retrieval system without written permission from the publisher, except for the inclusion of brief quotations in a review.

Blakkatz Publishing
Lincolnton, NC 28092

website: **http://www.blakkatz.com**
e-mail: **mbernard@blakkatz.com**

All Photographs © Michelle T. Bernard.

Note to the reader: This book is an informational guide. If you have questions regarding the health of your cat and possible problems related to diet or health, consult a professional veterinarian, preferably one who is listed with the Academy of Veterinary Homeopathy, **http://www.theavh.org** *or by telephone 866-652-1590.*

Library of Congress Cataloging-in-Publication Data

Bernard, Michelle T.

> Raising Cats Naturally: How to care for your cat the way nature intended/ Michelle T. Bernard – 1st ed.
> p. cm.
> Includes bibliographical references and index.
> ISBN 1-4276-0534-3
> 1.Cats. 2.Cats — Health. 3.Cats — Feeding and Feeds.

*This book is for Wiley, the most wonderful
creature in cat clothing to have
blessed my life — you left me too soon but
your spirit sat on my shoulder and helped
me to finish this book*

*"No one's death comes to pass without making some impression,
and those close to the deceased inherit part of
the liberated soul and become richer in their humaneness."
-- Richard Oxton Bolt*

Acknowledgment

Thanks to my good friends who have done nothing but encourage me throughout the writing and publishing of this book. A special thank you to all the people who assisted with the proof reading and the people who sent me their stories for inclusion in this book.

To those people on the Internet who challenged me – thank you. It was you who forced me to dig deeper and study feline nutrition.

Thanks to all the members of the Natural Cat List at Yahoo Groups who gave me the opportunity to learn from their experiences – and you all thought you were learning from me!

Finally, thanks to my cats, past and present – they taught me how to care for them the way nature intended.

> *There is no distinction between friend and foe. It is important to treat them the same. Your enemy is your teacher.*
> *-- Gyalsay Rinpoche*

A Word from the Author

This is not intended as a "my way" diet or method of caring for cats. If I have learned nothing else over these years, it is that there are many ways to do things. I do not know everything. I do not want to know everything. That would be an enormous amount of responsibility.

> *"One who is too insistent on his own views finds few to agree with him."*
> *— Lao-Tzu*

This book is heavy in nutritional facts and information. I believe nutrition is one of the most important things in caring for a cat. If fed a proper diet, most cats will remain quite healthy throughout their lives. You may never need to use any of the health care information provided in this book. You can skim over the nutrition facts and figures and go back to them if necessary. I did not want to leave anything out and hope I have answered any questions you may have. If your veterinarian questions the diet you are feeding, this book can prepare you with the answers.

At one point in my life, I did feel there was a right way, a wrong way, and my way. I thought I knew everything. That was a miserable existence. Somehow, I got on the right path. I learned humility, gained courage, and found serenity. I could not be happier with my life today, even with its various difficulties. Today I accept life on life's terms and try not to be attached to my beliefs.

There was a time when this book was supposed to be a memoir based on my experiences in raising cats naturally. What a glorified sense of self-importance I once had. Who would want to read a story about me? I certainly am not that important nor am I famous! What I can do and what I hope I have done with this book is to share my knowledge and my experiences. The more cats and their caregivers I can help the happier it makes me.

This journey has been a learning experience. My cats have taught me a tremendous amount. I am comfortable with how I have cared for them, even during those dark years. They have been able to hold on to their natural heritage as obligate carnivores and highly spiritual creatures.

> *The souls of pure teachers are arriving like rays of sunlight from so far up to the ground-huggers."*
> *— Rumi*

Using natural rearing methods has enabled me to bond with my cats on a far deeper level than I believe is possible for most feline caretakers. I do not use the word "owner" throughout this book. No one has the right to own another living being.

The effort I put into making my cats' food and their care is almost a second job. There are many times I wish I did not have to spend those hours cutting up meat and mixing supplement, but I could not imagine doing it any differently.

There is no right way or wrong way to care for cats, but if you want to keep your cat true to his birthright, this is how I found you can do it. I believe your cat will thank you for it and you will be blessed to share your life with a truly magnificent creature.

Michelle Bernard
Lincolnton, NC

Disclaimer

In this book I am sharing with you what I have learned over the years in caring for and feeding my cats. They have all done extremely well eating a raw meat diet, no matter what the formulation. In light of the research I have conducted, I believe the diet detailed in this book is sound and nutritionally complete for cats of all ages.

If you have an ill cat you should check with a veterinarian, preferably a holistic veterinarian, before switching to a raw meat diet. I will caution you that most conventional veterinarians will not agree with feeding a raw meat diet to your cat. Please keep in mind that most veterinarians, even those who label themselves as "holistic," received their training in feline nutrition from representatives of pet food companies. Unless they elected to pursue additional study in feline nutrition, this is most likely all the training they received. Conventional veterinarians are taught how to treat disease, not how to prevent it. Proper nutrition is a powerful tool in prevention of disease. The adage "you are what you eat" is so true when it is applied to a cat.

Pet food manufacturers want to sell their product. They advertise their food as being 100 percent nutritionally complete. I beg to differ. In the almost ten years I have been feeding a raw meat diet to my numerous cats, they have remained virtually free from the chronic disease that so plagues cats these days. Coincidence? I do not think so.

I suggest you research on your own the various commercial foods available and then look at how cats have evolved as predators. They are obligate carnivores that are designed to eat other animals. I believe you should feed your cat the way nature intended.

Contents

Chapter 1 – Early Lessons in Proper Feeding From Pottenger's Cats 1
Chapter 2 - Why Feed Raw? 4
    The Relationship Between Chronic Disease and Commercial Cat Food 4
Chapter 3 – Understanding the Basics of Feeding a Carnivore 8
    AAFCO and Animal Testing 8
    Other Raw Diets 10
Chapter 4 - Protein 12
    Table 1 - Protein and Fat Content of Various Wild Animals 12
    Table 2 - An analysis of a wild rabbit recipe compared to a chicken thigh recipe 14
    Table 3 - An analysis of a wild rabbit recipe compared to a turkey leg recipe 15
    Table 4 - An analysis of a wild rabbit recipe compared to a beef recipe 17
    Pork 18
    Fish 18
    Emergency Rations 19
Chapter 5 - Bone and Grinding 21
    Analysis of Copper and Zinc in Various Meats 21
    Bone and its relationship to constipation 22
    Grinding 27
    Commercially-prepared raw meat for pets 28
    Dental health 30
    Chicken or turkey necks 31
    The beauty of raw meat 31
Chapter 6 - Amino Acids 33
    Taurine 33
    Table 5 - An analysis of 200 grams of raw chicken heart 33
    Table 6 - Taurine Content in Various Foods 35
    Mixing Proteins 36
    Arginine 36
    Miscellaneous amino acids 37
Chapter 7 - Fats and Fatty Acids 38
Chapter 8 - Organ Meat 41
    Table 7 - An analysis of 100 grams of raw chicken liver 41
    Table 8 – An Analysis of vitamin A in a sample recipe using chicken 42
Chapter 9 - Feeding Prey Animals – "Prey Night" 44
Chapter 10 - Variety 45
Chapter 11 - Carbohydrates and Fiber 46
    Table 9 – a Breakdown of Fiber and Carbohydrates in Popular Vegetables ... 49
    Fiber 50
Chapter 12 - Parasites and Other Nasties 52
    Salmonella and Eschericia coli 52

Table 10 – Intestinal Lengths of a Dog, Cat and Human 53
Toxoplasmosis 54

Chapter 13 - Diet Polish – Supplements to Round Out the Balance 56
Water 56
Egg Yolk 57
Psyllium Husk Powder 58
Salmon Oil 59
Kelp and Dulse 59
Table 9 - Nutritional Analysis of Various Sea Vegetables 60
Bone Meal 60
Gelatin 61
Glandulars 61
Vitamin E 61
Vitamin B 62

Chapter 14 - Recipe With Bone 63
Chapter 15 - Recipe Without Bone 65
Chapter 16 - Time Saving Tips 67
Chapter 17 - Serving Tips 69
Chapter 18 - Switching Reluctant Cats 72
Chapter 19 - Success Stories 77
Chapter 20 – Homeopathy 86
Miasms 90
How do homeopathic remedies work? 91
Where do homeopathic remedies come from? 93
How to Find a Homeopathic Veterinarian 94
Buying Homeopathic Remedies 96
How to Administer a Homeopathic Remedy 97

Chapter 21 – The Litter Box 99
Chapter 22 - The Scratching Post 103
Chapter 23 - Vaccination 104
A word of caution 106
Nosodes 108

Chapter 24 - Natural Health Care Tips 110
Upper Respiratory Infections 110
Ringworm 115
Other Minor Skin Problems 119
Fleas 122
Ear Mites 123
Trauma 124
Vomiting, Diarrhea and Constipation 127
Spaying/Neutering 131
Pregnancy and Delivery 132

Chapter 25 - Conclusion 136

Chapter 26 - Shopping List and Resources 137
Chapter 27 – Recommended Reading 140

Chapter 1 – Early Lessons in Proper Feeding From Pottenger's Cats

The findings from a ten-year feeding study of cats conducted a little over 70 years ago by a doctor in California reveal that feeding cats raw food had a dramatic and positive impact on their health and well-being when compared to cats fed cooked meat. Between 1932 and 1942, Francis M. Pottenger, Jr., M.D. researched the use of adrenal hormones in respiratory complaints such as asthma. Because cats cannot live without their adrenal glands they were used as laboratory animals to standardize the extracts. Pottenger maintained his cats on what was considered to be a high quality, nutritionally complete feline diet. The cats were fed *cooked* meat scraps (consisting of liver, tripe, sweetbreads, brains, heart and muscle) from a local sanatorium, raw milk and cod liver oil. Commercial cat food did not appear on the markets until the 1960's. In Pottenger's time, domestic cats either hunted for their food or were fed table scraps.[1]

Compared to the stainless steel cages laboratory cats live in today, Pottenger's cats dwelt in agreeable quarters. They lived in large outdoor pens overlooking the San Gabriel Valley. The outdoor area was covered with chicken wire for adequate sun exposure. They had a trench filled with clean sand for a litter box. The back of the pens was sheltered and contained a wooden floor and bedding. Caretakers removed the cats' uneaten meat and bones and cleaned and refilled the water containers daily.[2]

Even though they received such good care, Pottenger could not understand why the cats were such poor operative risks. Many died in surgery or recovered slowly.[3]

When the cats donated to Pottenger's study outnumbered the food available from the sanatorium, Pottenger placed an order at a local meat packing plant for *raw* meat scraps, again including the viscera, muscle and bone.[4]

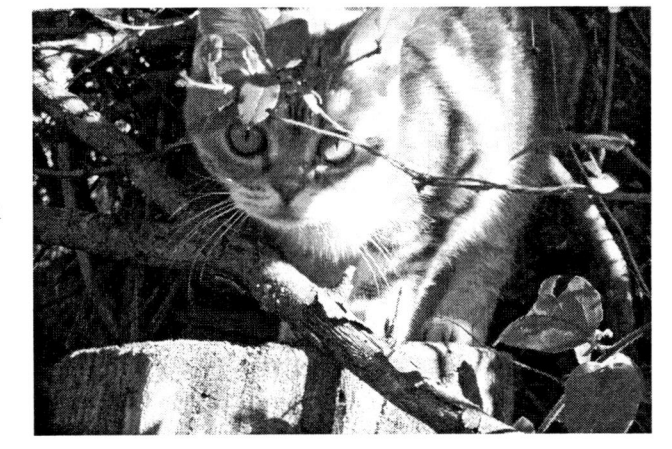

Pottenger fed the raw meat scraps (including raw milk and cod liver oil) to a segregated group of cats, keeping the remainder of his cats on the cooked meat diet. Within a few months the differences between the cats fed raw meat and those fed cooked meat became evident. The raw meat fed cats and kittens were more vigorous and survived surgery better than the cooked meat fed cats.[5]

The difference between the health of the two groups of cats prompted Pottenger to conduct a ten year study involving over 900 cats including at least four generations to discover why cats fed raw food were healthier than those fed cooked food. The cats in Pottenger's study were used to study the effects of heat-processed food to benefit human nutrition. The latest and most rigorous scientific standards were applied for these experiments with their protocol consistently observed. Each cat's clinical chart included notes for its entire life. At the end of ten years, 600 of 900 the cats studied had complete, recorded health histories.[6]

The raw meat fed cats were uniform in size and skeletal development from generation to generation. Over their life spans, they were resistant to infections, fleas and various other parasites and had no signs of allergies. In general, they were gregarious, friendly and predictable in their behavior patterns. They reproduced one homogeneous generation after another with the average weight of the kittens at birth being 119 grams (4.20 ounces). Miscarriages were rare and litters averaged five kittens with the mother cat nursing her young without difficulty.[7]

The cats fed the cooked meat diet reproduced a heterogeneous strain of offspring, each kitten in a litter different in size and skeletal pattern. Health problems ranged from allergies to infections of the kidney, liver, bones and reproductive organs. By the time the third deficient generation was born, the cats were so "physiologically bankrupt" that none survived beyond sixth months, thus terminating the strain.[8]

Cooked meat fed cats showed much more irritability. Some females were dangerous to handle. The males, on the other hand, were docile, often unassertive and lacked sex drive or were perverted.[9]

Pregnant females aborted, about 25 percent in the first deficient generation to about 70 percent in the second generation. Deliveries were generally difficult with many females dying in labor. Kittens' mortality rate was also high because they were either stillborn or too frail to nurse.[10]

Many females had pregnancy and infertility problems. The average weight of the kittens born of cooked meat fed mothers was 100 grams (3.4 ounces), 19 grams less than the raw meat nurtured kittens.[11]

Raw-meat fed males of proven virility were used for breeding, therefore, the experimental results primarily reflected the condition of the mother cat.[12]

Most deficient cats died from infections of the kidneys, lungs and bones.[13] If modern-day antibiotics had been applied, these infections would possibly have been eliminated as a cause of death. The use of antibiotics to treat infections would have allowed the cats to reveal their ultimate degenerative fates.

Many of the deficiencies experienced by the cats fed the cooked meat diet were due to inadequate taurine. Cooking meat makes taurine less available to cats. Pottenger's study demonstrates that cats thrived and reproduced for years on a very simple raw food diet.

With the advent of commercial cat food, scientists employed by pet food manufacturers conducted feed trials to determine the minimum daily requirements for the domestic cat. Laboratory cats, kept in small stainless steel cages, are fed a purified diet with different nutrients withheld until a deficiency emerges. With the Pottenger Cat Study records available, pet food manufacturers did not need to conduct their own feed trials. Pottenger's raw meat fed cats survived for years without the need for veterinary care. Why would there be a need to feed a cat any differently? Where did the public lose its way in feeding cats?

Chapter 2 - Why Feed Raw?

Let us take a closer look at commercial cat food.

The Relationship Between Chronic Disease and Commercial Cat Food

Many chronic diseases in cats can be directly associated with the now common practice of feeding commercial dry food to cats. These include dental disease, inflammatory bowel disease (IBD), feline urinary tract disorder, kidney disease, diabetes and probably even cancer. The correlation between the ingredients in commercial cat food and these diseases is too close to ignore.

> *"When the Earth is sick, the animals will begin to disappear, when that happens, the Warriors of the Rainbow will come to save them."*
> *-- Chief Seattle*

Take diabetes as an example. Male neutered cats older than six years old are most commonly diagnosed with diabetes and it is usually type 2. Obesity increases the risk for type 2 diabetes in cats fourfold.[14]

Type 2 diabetes is one of the most common feline endocrinopathies affecting 1 in 300 cats[15]. In her paper on feline diabetes, Dr. Deborah Greco states that, as with humans, the best approach to treatment of cats with Type 2 diabetes is diet and exercise.[16] She suggests one way of increasing a diabetic cat's activity is to hide meals in various places throughout the house. I vote for letting a couple of mice loose in the house and letting the cat chase them.

The cat as an obligate carnivore is unique in its insulin response to dietary carbohydrates, protein and fat. Amino acids, rather than glucose, signal insulin release in cats.[17] Normal cats maintain essential glucose requirements from amino acids rather than from dietary carbohydrates.[18] As a result, cats can maintain normal blood glucose concentrations even when deprived of food for over 72 hours. *The cat is uniquely adapted to a carnivorous diet (mice) and is not metabolically adapted to ingestion of excess carbohydrate.*[19]

Most commercial cat food is extremely high in carbohydrates, thereby predisposing cats to obesity and diabetes.

Many cats with IBD enjoy a complete reversal of symptoms when they are taken entirely off commercial food and fed a diet similar to the one in this book.

A 1995 study conducted by the National Companion Animal Study concluded that oral disease was the most common feline ailment.[20] Could this be due to the commercial food they consume? In his book, *Variations and Diseases of the*

Teeth of Animals, Colyer examined 1,157 wild canid skulls and reported the periodontal diseases as suggested by alveolar bone destruction was present in only 2 percent of the specimens.[21]

Typical dry dog and cat foods contribute little dental cleansing. As a tooth penetrates a kibble or treat the initial contact causes the food to shatter and crumble with contact only at the coronal tip of the tooth surface.[22] *The general belief that dry foods provide significant oral cleansing should be regarded with skepticism.* A moist food may perform similarly to a typical dry food in affecting plaque, stain and calculus accumulation.[23]

The stimulus for thirst appears to be less sensitive in cats than in dogs. Cats are able to survive on less water than dogs and may ignore minor levels of dehydration. Cats compensate for reduced water intake, in part, by forming highly concentrated urine which predisposes them to feline lower urinary tract disease (FLUTD).[24] Consumption of dry food increases the risk for lower urinary tract disease in cats.[25] This makes complete sense. Cats evolved as desert creatures – if need be, they could remain hydrated solely from their food source. A mouse is 65-75 percent moisture. Dry food is less than 10 percent moisture; a cat needs to drink a considerable amount of water to remain hydrated. Some cats do not care to drink water so they remain in a constant state of dehydration. Dry food is often left constantly available to cats. Increased frequency of feeding is associated with an increased risk of urinary tract disease, regardless of food. Obese and inactive cats are at increased risk as well.[26]

> *"Speak the truth in a million voices. It is silence that kills."*
> *– Catherine of Sienna*

I have lost track of how many different formulas Iams and Science Diet are marketing these days. I know both companies are deeply entrenched in the prescription diet market. Prescription foods are for cats and dogs that get sick while eating the regular formulas. You can no longer count on one type of cat food take your cat through all stages of her life. You can start with kitten food, then once your kitten reaches a magical age and becomes an adult you can switch to adult food. Perhaps you will feed adult food for a few years, then you

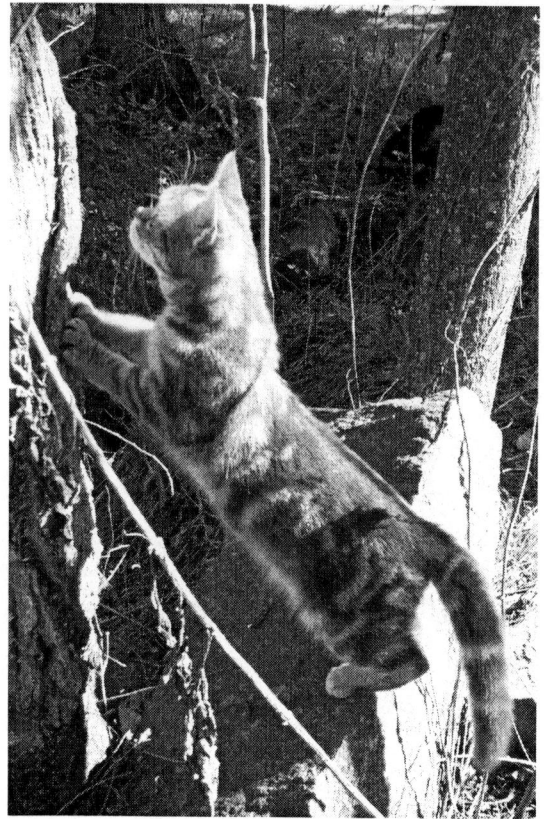

may need to switch to an obesity formula (if your cat gets too fat on the adult formula), a dental diet (if your cat develops dental problems while on the adult cat food), a sensitive formula (if your cat develops skin or stomach problems while eating the adult cat food), one of the many different lower urinary tract formulas (if your cat develops feline urologic syndrome [FUS], oxalate crystals or struvite crystals), a heart formula (if your cat develops a heart condition) and so on. Where does it end – when your cat dies? Then it starts over with the next kitten. It is a terribly vicious cycle.

Commercial cat food, especially dry cat food, is not healthy for most cats. If it were, why would so many different formulas be necessary? If their food was truly 100 percent nutritionally balanced and complete, would there be such a need for all the prescription foods? In all the years I have been feeding raw to my cats, I have not had to change the formulation of the diet I feed them to address an illness.

Dry food in particular is unhealthy for cats, no matter what formula, shape, texture, packaging or how clever the marketing. The two major problems with dry food is the lack of moisture and the excessive carbohydrate content. Dry food is cooked and processed to death. Dry food bears as little resemblance to meat as potato chips do to potatoes. At least most potato chips contain *potatoes*. It is hard to find a dry cat food that contains just *chicken*, you have chicken, chicken meal, chicken by-product, poultry by-product, chicken flavor and chicken digest. Would you buy potato chips that listed potato by-product or potato digest as an ingredient?

Canned food is usually not much better than dry in ingredient quality, but at least it contains sufficient water. Canned cat foods generally have moisture contents above 60 percent moisture. That is a great benefit for your cat! Cats should be getting their moisture from their food. Dry food is more economical than canned food and of course easier to feed.

I believe all commercial cat food is inferior to a raw diet like the one detailed in this book, but if you cannot take the time to feed raw, then feed a canned food that contains human grade *meat* (not by-product) and contains minimal, if any, grains. There are such foods available.

You will see throughout this book the cat is referred to as an "obligate carnivore." The cat is a member of order *Carnivora*. Cats and other members of the superfamily *Feloidea* are considered obligate carnivores as they have strict requirements for certain nutrients that can only be found in animal tissues. Cats cannot synthesize taurine or arginine, amino acids found only in meat. They lack the ability to convert linoleic acid (contain in plants) to arachidonic acid (contained in animal fat). They cannot convert beta-carotene to vitamin A. Cats cannot decrease activity of hepatic enzymes when fed low-protein foods – they must consume a high protein diet. Cats must eat meat to survive.

I cannot believe anyone can really look at these different cat foods and feel confident feeding them. What is the right formula? protein? grain? shape? I know many breeders who mix several different types of dry food together because they do not trust just one brand fed alone to be nutritionally complete. That causes problems itself because if a cat develops intolerance to one brand (and they do that regularly), you do not know which brand it is because you are feeding several different brands.

It makes so much more sense to prepare a balanced raw meat diet and feed that to your cats. It is what a cat, an animal that is an obligate carnivore, is supposed to eat. It should be fed to them raw. No animal cooks its food in the wild. It should be fed in as close to its natural state as possible. It should contain ingredients as high quality as the caregiver can afford. It should be fresh. It should be served with love and respect for the animal you are feeding.

"This is the miracle that happens every time to
those who really love; the more they give, the more they possess."
-- Rainer Maria Rilke

Chapter 3 – Understanding the Basics of Feeding a Carnivore

The diet portion of this book presents a detailed explanation of how to prepare a homemade diet consisting of raw meat and supplements. For purposes of this book, the term "recipe" shall mean approximately 1,000 grams of meat, bone and organ meat, water, egg yolks and supplements. The recipe is very similar in ingredients and proportions to the one presented in Feline Future's *The Backyard Predator*.[27] Feline Future did a wonderful job constructing a raw diet using minimal species-appropriate ingredients.

I believe you should know *why* a particular ingredient is in the recipe before you know how much. Therefore, the recipes are included at the end of the diet section.

AAFCO and Animal Testing

Minimum nutritional requirements for cats have been compiled by the Association of American Feed Control Officials (AAFCO) and various other entities. These data were compiled under laboratory or other artificial conditions. I do not condone the use of cats or any other animal as laboratory subjects. I believe that in many instances, the testing done on dogs and cats by the pet food industry is as bad as the testing done by the medical and cosmetic industries. Keep in mind if you are feeding commercial food – that some poor cat may have suffered through some terrible experiment conducted by the manufacturer. Poor quality aside, that is reason enough in my mind *not* to feed commercial cat food. No cats suffered during the creation and testing of this diet.

I do not believe these laboratory tests take into account the true nature of the cat as a predator and obligate carnivore. What is necessary to keep a cat alive in a stainless steel laboratory cage is of no interest to me. What keeps cats *healthy* under conditions similar to how they would live naturally is the true indicator. I discovered early on that keeping neutered and spayed cats healthy using a raw diet was quite easy. It is a true art to keep breeding and show cats healthy on a raw diet. What keeps a pregnant cat and ultimately her kittens healthy and in good condition is a diet that is truly nutritionally balanced and species-appropriate.

Pregnant cats, kittens, adults and older cats all eat essentially the same food in the wild. There are no sensitive stomach or hairball reduction mice – they are not necessary. The prey a wild cat catches and eats is perfect nutrition for all stages of life. No modification is needed except for frequency in eating. My pregnant cats, weaning kittens and senior cats all eat exactly the same food. They always have.

I have been feeding a raw meat diet to my cats since 1993. I am glad I discovered raw feeding by accident instead of how so many people do now, when their cats are so sick they are drawn to a raw diet in a last ditch attempt to heal their cat. Please, once you realize the potential dangers associated with feeding a commercial diet, do not feel guilty!

> *"Learn to trust your own judgment, learn inner independence, learn to trust that time will sort good from bad – including your own bad."*
> — Doris Lessing

I purchased *The New Natural Cat* by Anitra Frazier to fulfill a Book of the Month Club membership. I had no interest in natural cat care at the time. After I read the chapter on diet, I realized I was doing my cats a lot of harm in "free-feeding" (leaving food out for them to graze on all day) commercial dry food. I immediately took away the dry food and purchased a natural canned food and the supplements recommended in the book. It took a day and a half for Rooney to adapt to the new diet. Pumpkin refused to touch it. It took me almost five months to get Pumpkin to accept her new diet. It was Pumpkin's refusal to eat that led me to explore homeopathy. Homeopathy is a form of medicine developed by a doctor in Germany in the late 1700s.

Rooney began to show the effects of the new diet while I was trying to convince Pumpkin that I was not trying to poison her. Rooney had become a bit chubby while eating dry food. The excess fat dropped off and was replaced with muscle. His coat took on a wonderful shine and I began to notice less shedding, an increase in activity level and less litter box odor. I took a further step and started feeding a completely homemade diet consisting of human-grade raw meat, cooked grains and vegetables, raw garlic, parsley and carrots, a vitamin/mineral supplement and oils.

Since 1993, my clan has grown considerably and Blakkatz Cattery was born. I have streamlined my production of the diet so it takes very little time. I continue to see excellent benefits from feeding a homemade diet.

Initially I used a diet developed by Jeffrey Levy, a homeopathic veterinarian living in Williamsburg, Massachusetts.[28] This was an extremely complex diet with a lot of ingredients. As I learned more about a natural feline diet, my diet evolved to what it is today.

> *"The time you spend preparing your cat's meals, the personal energy you put into it, is a gift of great value and a true measure of your love"*
> — *Jeffrey Levy, D.V.M.*

Other Raw Diets

At one time I was worried about my diet changing - was I ever feeding the wrong food or an unbalanced diet to my cats? Dr. Levy's diet, Anitra Frazier's diet (*The New Natural Cat*) and Dr. Pitcairn's diets are all far better than feeding a commercial diet. The problem with all of these diets is that they are not taking into account what you are feeding – a small cat. The cat evolved as an obligate carnivore. All of the above diets include ingredients like grains, vegetables, garlic, yeast, vitamin C, and alfalfa. While these additions may be good for humans, they are not necessarily good for cats and may be harmful. There are still many raw diets available on the Internet and in natural cat care books that recommend garlic, vegetables, vitamin C and so forth. I do not think they are necessary or desirable. I do not feed these ingredients to my cats.

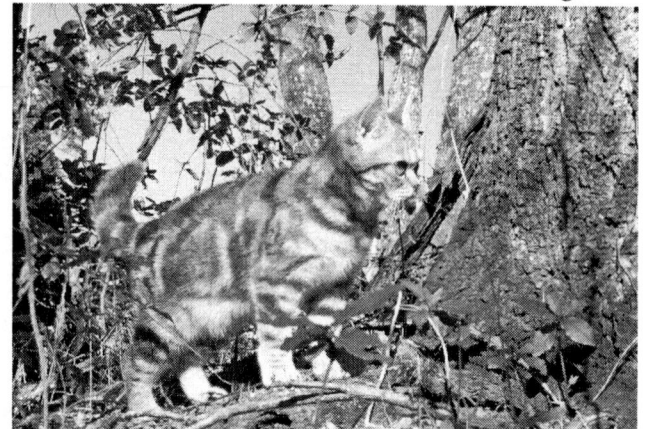

For example, a cat's natural diet has little or no vitamin C. Meat has little or no vitamin C. Cats can manufacture their own vitamin C. If vitamin C is not abundant in their natural prey, why should it be added to a homemade diet? The same argument can be applied to garlic. As far as I know even the mice in Italy are garlic-free. Why add garlic to your cat food -- because it is supposed to be a natural antibiotic or flea deterrent? Even if that were so, a healthy cat will not need antibiotics of any kind and should not become infested with fleas. It just does not make sense. More importantly, cats usually do not like the taste of garlic. Why add something to their food if they do not like it?

New Age ingredients like garlic, aloe, yucca and chicory are showing up in commercial cat foods to make the cat food appear healthy and natural to the consumer. Long-term use of ingredients such as garlic may be detrimental to a cat. Garlic or any member of the onion family can cause a cat's red blood cells to malfunction and which in turn causes a condition known as Heinz Body Anemia. Garlic is listed as a poison to cats and to some extent, dogs on the ASPCA poison control web site.[29]

Addition of vitamin C, tomato, cranberries, or other acidic ingredients is not necessary. A cat eating a natural diet of rat carcasses maintains an average urinary pH of 6.3.[30] It does not take any more than that – feed a cat a species-appropriate diet and all is well.

Chapter 4 - Protein

Meat or protein (meaning muscle meat, bone, organ meat and egg yolks) is the most important part of this diet. Meat is where you should focus your attention and put your money. The ideal meat to feed your cat is rabbit, as Yukon is eating in the photograph on this page, or other game animals. I do not advocate hunting for pleasure or sport; however, if you know someone who hunts ethically, be very nice to him and hope that he'll provide you with fresh killed

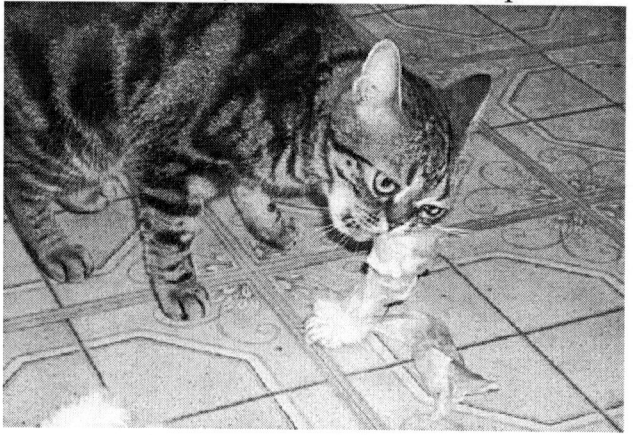

rabbit, squirrel, or venison. Even though a small wild cat would not kill a deer, venison has the same protein to fat ratios and is nutritionally close to prey that a cat would naturally eat. Table 1 demonstrates that grazing animals living in their natural state are leaner and have a higher protein content than animals that are raised conventionally.

Table 1 - Protein and Fat Content of Various Wild Animals

Animal (100 g)	Moisture (g)	Protein (g)	Fat (g)	Cholesterol (mg)
Buffalo	74.5	21.7	1.9	62
Whitetail Deer	73.5	23.6	1.4	116
Mule Deer	73.4	23.7	1.3	107
Elk	74.8	22.8	0.9	87
Moose	75.8	22.1	0.5	71
Antelope	73.9	22.5	0.9	112
Squirrel	73.8	21.4	3.2	83
Cottontail	74.5	21.8	2.4	77
Jackrabbit	73.8	21.9	2.4	131
Wild Turkey	71.7	25.7	1.1	55
Wild Pheasant	72.4	25.7	0.6	52
Grey Partridge	72.1	25.6	0.7	85
Sharptail Grouse	74.2	23.8	0.7	105
Sage Grouse	74.3	23.7	1.1	101
Dove	73.8	22.9	1.8	94
Sandhill Crane	73.2	21.7	2.4	123

Animal (100 g)	Moisture (g)	Protein (g)	Fat (g)	Cholesterol (mg)
Snow Goose	71.1	22.7	3.6	142
Mallard	73.2	23.1	2.0	140
Widgeon	73.5	22.6	2.1	131

*grams per 100 grams
**milligrams per 100 grams

Cooperative Extension Service
University of Illinois

Grazing animals eating their natural food (grass) also have higher levels of vitamin E and omega 3 fatty acids in their tissues.[31]

Wild cats kill and eat rabbits. Often, rabbit is their primary prey.[32] In my analysis comparing various types of meat available to make cat food, I recommend a recipe of 700 grams of raw wild rabbit, 2 raw egg yolks, 200 grams of raw chicken heart and 100 grams of raw chicken liver as the "goal" you should strive for. Unfortunately, because it is not a common food for humans, I was unable to find an analysis for rabbit liver or heart so I substituted chicken.

The various analysis tables I have provided are for muscle meat only. It is assumed with chicken or rabbit you will grind the meat with the bone. There is considerable fat in bone marrow which will raise the total fat content of the diet. Also, if you can source rabbit or chicken with their heads intact, use the heads. The contents of the head (nerve tissues like the brain, eyes [optic nerves and retina] and spinal cord) provide valuable nutrients (such as taurine) for your cat. Perhaps that is why cats usually eat their mice headfirst.[33]

In Table 2, I compared the wild rabbit recipe to a recipe consisting of 700 grams of raw skinless chicken thigh, 200 grams chicken heart, 100 grams chicken liver and two raw egg yolks. You will see chicken thigh is reasonably close in nutritional value to wild rabbit. The chicken thigh recipe, even though it is skinless, is lower in protein and higher in fat than wild rabbit.

Table 2 - An analysis of a wild rabbit recipe compared to a chicken thigh recipe

Nutrient	700 grams raw wild rabbit, 200 grams raw chicken heart, 100 grams raw chicken liver, and two raw egg yolks	700 grams raw skinless chicken thigh, 200 grams raw chicken heart, 100 grams raw chicken liver and two raw egg yolks
Calories	1347.86	1382.86
Pro (g)	207.38	192.68
Fat (g)	48.86	60.06
Carb (g)	5.4	5.4
Fiber (g)	0	0
Cal (mg)	164.48	150.48
Iron (mg)	44.16	28.76
Na (mg)	591.28	843.28
Pot (mg)	3257.21	2228.21
Phos (mg)	2370.02	1964.02
Ash (g)	11.3	10.6
vitA(IU)	21254.74	21709.74
vitC (mg)	40.2	61.9
Thia (mg)	0.71	1.03
Ribo (mg)	4.05	4.95
Nia (mg)	64.52	63.33
H2O percent	67.63	67.95
satF (g)	14.62	16.79
monoF (g)	14	18.06
polyF (g)	10.6	14.24
Chol (mg)	1703.29	1717.29

Analysis completed using the Nutritional Analysis Tool 2.0 **http://www.nat.uiuc.edu**

This is a perfect illustration of the differences in nutritional value of a conventionally raised animal as compared to a wild animal. There is not much you can do about these nutritional variations unless you are going to take up hunting. I realize I'm comparing a bird to a mammal, but if you look at Table 1, the fat content of small birds is even less than the jackrabbit.

You can compensate for the deficiencies in minerals like iron, niacin and potassium by adding kelp and dulse to the recipe. Interestingly, the 5.4 grams of carbohydrates came from the chicken heart and liver. Use of raw ground bone will change the calcium to phosphorus (Ca:P) ratios substantially as well as many of the mineral figures. An analysis of kelp, dulse, nori, and alaria is shown on Table 9.

If you use chicken breast with the skin, the protein and fat ratios will be closer, but since chicken leg meat is higher in taurine and fat than chicken breast meat, it is better to use chicken legs on a more frequent basis than chicken breast.[34] Chicken leg is usually less expensive than breast. You can substitute chopped up chicken breast with the bone (with no supplements) a meal or two a week to add variety.

The use of whole chicken brings the chicken values even closer to wild rabbit. While I sometimes use whole chickens, it is a considerable amount of work cutting the chicken into pieces small enough to run through the feed tube of a meat grinder. It is also a lot harder getting the skin off whole chickens. If you are handy with a knife or kitchen shears, whole chicken is the best. Use the organ meat that comes with the bird in addition to what is added to the recipe.

As you will see from Table 3, skinless turkey leg including organ meat and eggs is closer to wild rabbit meat than chicken. The problem with using turkey versus chicken is handling the bone. Turkey thigh bone if crushed with a heavy cleaver will go through the Maverick grinder. Turkey drumstick bone will not. In my experience, the only affordable grinder that will handle turkey bones is the Tasin TS-108, which at one time was sold by Northern Tool. See the sourcing guide for where to purchase this grinder. If in doubt, hack it up. This makes a huge mess and you need to be pretty handy with a cleaver to do it. Your work area will end up looking like a scene from Texas Chainsaw Massacre. Keep chanting, "It's for the good of my cats. It's for the good of my cats," and you will get through it. If using turkey means you cannot grind the bone, then stick to chicken and feed turkey on an occasional basis.

Table 3 - An analysis of a wild rabbit recipe compared to a turkey leg recipe

Nutrient	700 grams raw wild rabbit, 200 grams raw chicken heart, 100 grams raw chicken liver, and two raw egg yolks	700 grams raw skinless turkey thigh, 200 grams raw chicken heart, 100 grams raw chicken liver and two raw egg yolks
Calories	1347.86	1305.86
Pro (g)	207.38	197.58
Fat (g)	48.86	49.56
Carb (g)	5.4	5.4
Fiber (g)	0	0
Cal (mg)	164.48	150.48
Iron (mg)	44.16	34.36

Nutrient	700 grams raw wild rabbit, 200 grams raw chicken heart, 100 grams raw chicken liver, and two raw egg yolks	700 grams raw skinless turkey thigh, 200 grams raw chicken heart, 100 grams raw chicken liver and two raw egg yolks
Na (mg)	591.28	738.28
Pot (mg)	3257.21	2389.21
Phos (mg)	2370.02	1992.02
Ash (g)	11.3	9.9
vitA (IU)	21254.74	21254.74
vitC (mg)	40.2	40.2
Thia (mg)	0.71	0.85
Ribo (mg)	4.05	5.1
Nia (mg)	64.52	37.78
H2O percent	67.63	68.15
satF (g)	14.62	15.39
monoF (g)	14	13.37
polyF (g)	10.6	12.42
Chol (mg)	1703.29	1724.29

Analysis completed using the Nutritional Analysis Tool 2.0 **http://www.nat.uiuc.edu**

A combination of raw conventionally-raised beef, beef heart, beef liver and raw egg yolks is quite different than the wild rabbit model shown in Table 4. Beef is far lower in protein and much higher in fat, especially saturated fat. I normally advise against feeding conventionally raised beef to cats. Many cats, especially those new to raw or with IBD, cannot tolerate beef. The ratio of omega 6 to omega 3 fatty acid of conventionally raised beef is 5:1 to 13:1 compared to 2:1 in grass-fed beef.[35] Cattle are customarily butchered at about two years of age. By that time, a significant amount of toxins may have accumulated in the cow's fat.[36] Cattle are routinely given antibiotics, growth hormones and often fed grain containing rendered animals (containing even more accumulated toxins). Conventional meat production is producing unhealthy animals. They are not particularly healthy for anyone to eat. If you can source grass-fed beef or beef that is naturally raised at a reasonable price, that would be a better option to feed your cat. Grass-fed beef is comparable to wild game in their protein to fat and omega 6 to omega 3 fatty acid ratios.[37]

Conventionally raised chicken is not much better than beef, but you can remove the skin and cut out a good deal of the fat. Organic or naturally raised chicken is usually less expensive than organic beef. If necessary, locate a wholesale source for organic chicken and buy it by the case to cut down the expense.

Table 4 - An analysis of a wild rabbit recipe compared to a beef recipe

Nutrient	700 grams raw wild rabbit, 200 grams raw chicken heart, 100 grams raw chicken liver, and two raw egg yolks	700 grams raw beef, 200 grams raw beef heart, 100 grams raw beef liver and two raw egg yolks
Calories	1347.86	2532.86
Pro (g)	207.38	180.88
Fat (g)	48.86	190.46
Carb (g)	5.4	11.6
Fiber (g)	0	0
Cal (mg)	164.48	111.48
Iron (mg)	44.16	29.76
Na (mg)	591.28	626.28
Pot (mg)	3257.21	2755.21
Phos (mg)	2370.02	1904.02
Ash (g)	11.3	9.5
vitA(IU)	21254.74	35991.74
vitC (mg)	40.2	34.6
Thia (mg)	0.71	1.26
Ribo (mg)	4.05	6.15
Nia (mg)	64.52	56.49
H2O percent	67.63	62.68
satF (g)	14.62	75.18
monoF (g)	14	79.38
polyF (g)	10.6	10.51
Chol (mg)	1703.29	1577.29

Analysis completed using the Nutritional Analysis Tool 2.0 **http://www.nat.uiuc.edu**

Some breeders supplement their cats' diets with raw beef to help keep good weight on them. They tend to use beef because they are afraid of salmonella from chicken. The beef that many breeders feed comes from companies that produce raw meat for pet food such as suppliers of meat for greyhound breeders. This meat is often from cows not fit for human consumption; for example, from cows that for one reason or another did not make it to the slaughterhouse alive (called "downed" cows). In addition, the FDA requires that meat sold for pets must be denatured, meaning a chemical – like charcoal is added to the meat to render it not fit for human consumption.

Given the analyses provided, it is evident why feeding your cat a diet of rabbit (if you can get it) or game meats (again, if you can source them), skinless chicken thighs, or turkey thighs is closer to what he would eat in the wild.

Meals of beef or lamb once in a while are fine, but I would not make beef or lamb the mainstay of your cat's diet. As mentioned above, many cats cannot tolerate beef or lamb. Before you make up an entire recipe of beef or lamb, offer a few pieces to your cat to see if it will stay down. Stew lamb or beef pieces make great chew toys or pseudo prey.

Pork

There is danger of your cat contracting trichinosis from raw pork. In addition, 100 grams of pork has 2.030 grams of saturated fat compared to 1.000 grams in chicken thigh and 0.690 grams in wild rabbit. I suggest that you do not feed raw pork.

"Pigs are magical, but not their flesh or bones!"
— Juliette de Bairacli Levy

Keep high fat meats to a minimum. Cats may like the taste of fat, but excessive fat, especially if it is from an animal fed grain, is not healthy for them. Your cat should be a lean, mean, fighting machine!

If you can obtain meat that has not been bled out, that is very beneficial for your cat. Do not drain the blood from the organ meat — add it right into the meat mixture. My feline vampires gather at the bowl when I prepare the diet to drink the blood at the bottom of the bowl from the heart and liver.

Fish

I feed fish once or twice a month. I usually use cans of Jack Mackerel, whole raw smelt, or raw catfish chunks. The problem with fish is that cats tend to like it too much. If it is fed too frequently, they may hold out for fish and not want meat. Do not feed fish to your cat if he has a history of urinary tract disorder. Fish is very high in magnesium: .039 percent compared to chicken muscle meat that is .013 percent.[38] These percentages are without bone. If you add in bone, the percentages would be higher as magnesium is the third largest mineral constituent of bone, after calcium and phosphorus. As a comparison, a mouse carcass (including bone) is approximately 0.16 percent magnesium.[39,40] An adult chicken carcass (including bone) is approximately 0.50 percent.[41,42] Excessive magnesium in the diet can lead to struvite urinary crystals, while a deficit has been shown to increase the risk of calcium oxalate urolithiasis in rats.[43]

Fish is a good food to add every once in a while for variety, but it should not be a staple food. When I feed fish, I feed it as it is (no supplements).

Emergency Rations

Some people new to feeding a raw diet express concern about an Act of Nature, coming home late from work, forgetting to thaw out food, or some other fiasco preventing them from feeding raw food to their cats. Many of these people keep canned food on hand for such instances. Canned food, especially a high-quality brand like Wysong, would be an acceptable short-term substitute, but feeding your cat processed food after he has been on raw for any length of time could cause stomach upset.

If you go away, even if it is just for a weekend, you will need to hire a pet sitter to come in twice a day to feed your cat. I believe a visit from a pet sitter twice a day is not out of line no matter what you are feeding your cat. Your cat is accustomed to you being there and he will miss you if you are gone. You do not know what sort of trouble your cat could get into while you are away and someone checking in could avert a disaster.

If you make the commitment to feed raw, you will definitely need to make arrangements for your cat to be fed and cared for at least twice a day when you are away. Do not think you can leave your raw-fed cat for a weekend with several bowls of dry food and a clean litter box. Switching a cat accustomed to eating raw food to dry food for the weekend will result in severe stomach upset and diarrhea.

> *"You become responsible forever for what you have tamed."*
> — *Antoine de Saint-Exupery*

If you come home late from work and have forgotten to take out food or you do not have it made up, you can use any of the following "emergency rations" to feed your cat. You do not need to resort to canned food.

- boneless chicken thighs;
- chicken breast with the bone;
- chicken necks;
- chopped up Cornish Game Hens;
- raw egg yolks or whole eggs;
- cottage cheese;
- canned mackerel;
- whole smelt;
- catfish chunks;
- beef or lamb stew meat;
- chopped-up beef heart;
- chopped-up beef kidney; or
- small lamb chops.

All of the above or anything similar can be fed without supplements once or twice a week. Use of the foods mentioned above will also help make up for any dietary deficiencies if you feed predominately poultry. Dairy products can cause stomach upset in some cats.

Chapter 5 - Bone and Grinding

The best thing about using rabbit, chicken, or turkey is that you will be able to grind meat with the bone – which is the way it should be done. Do not use bone meal or other calcium supplement unless you absolutely have to and not on a long-term basis. Bone is more than calcium! The actual form of calcium in bone is called "Hydroxyapatite." Other minerals in bone are: magnesium, zinc, manganese, copper, boron, silica, phosphorus, fluoride, sodium and potassium.[44]

One hundred grams of bone contain 25,000 mg calcium, 12,000 mg phosphorus, 370 mg magnesium, 700 mg potassium, 9 mg zinc and 0.5 mg copper.[45]

Chicken muscle meat is particularly low in copper and zinc. Feeding chicken muscle meat and using a calcium supplement may eventually result in a copper or zinc deficiency. Cheetahs fed a diet consisting primarily of chicken carcass suffered copper deficiencies.[46]

Analysis of Copper and Zinc in Various Meats

	Copper (mg/kg)	Zinc (mg/kg)
Chicken Muscle Meat (no bone)	0.41	9.3[47]
Chicken Carcass	3.6	116.1[48,49]
Adult Mouse Carcass	6.7	67.5[50,51]
Domestic Rabbit Carcass	4.6	84.0[52]

Around 30 percent of bone is composed of organic compounds, of which 90 to 95 percent is collagen the rest being non-collagenous proteins. Collagen is a fibrous protein that provides the bone with strength and flexibility. It is an important component of many other tissues, including skin and tendons. Collagen is comprised of many amino acids, including hydroxyproline and threonine (which helps prevent fat build-up in the liver, helps the digestive and intestinal tracts function more smoothly and assists metabolism and assimilation).

Gelatin is a substitute for collagen and various amino acids if you do not use raw bone. As you may know, gelatin is recommended for strong nails. I often wonder if the reason why my cats are "claw factories" is because they get so much raw collagen in their diets. It seems like I clip their claws and in no time they have grown new daggers.

One of the reasons why kelp and dulse are added to the recipe is to replace some of the minerals that are lost in bone meal by processing. Bone meal is cooked and processed. Ground raw bone is a thousand times better than bone meal or any other calcium substitute. Feeding a raw diet and using bone meal for any length of time could result in dietary deficiencies such as copper and zinc.

If you have been using meat without bone, you will be surprised to see how red even chicken is when you grind the bone. Think of all the goodness your cat is getting from the raw bone!

Bone and its relationship to constipation

There is some thought that raw bone or bone meal causes constipation in some cats. Excess calcium in the diet will cause constipation, however, using chicken legs or whole chickens with the bone is not excessive. I have not seen that. As of this writing, I am feeding nine cats ranging in age from nine months to twelve years old. The only constipation my cats had was due to illness or confinement. I believe frequent constipation, like frequent diarrhea, is a chronic illness that should be addressed using homeopathy, not by substituting another calcium supplement. I also believe people who are new to feeding a raw diet to their cats are used to a more voluminous, softer stool than what is normal for a cat fed a species-appropriate diet. A cat in the wild would not do well if he had to pass and bury cow plop stool several times a day.

Are we somehow creating a race of cats that cannot digest animal products? Is it a problem that is passing through the generations or is it due to excessive antibiotic use in kittens (antibiotics do cause intestinal disturbances), is it over-vaccination, or all of the above?

I have been hypothesizing for some time about commercial food causing the intestinal tract of cats to lengthen and lose tone and elasticity. This would result in both the diarrhea and constipation that has become quite chronic in cats of all ages. I can understand an older cat taken off a commercial food diet and put on a raw diet having constipation issues. The commercial diet would provide a great deal of bulk resulting in voluminous, soft stool. Bulky, soft stool passing through the cat's intestinal tract instead of more fibrous matter (such as bone and hide that is normal in a cat's natural diet) would, in my opinion, stretch the intestinal tract and cause it to lose elasticity. A properly balanced raw diet provides little bulk and contains mostly digestible ingredients resulting in little stool production. A cat should be digesting most of the food he consumes. I find it difficult to accept a young cat on a raw diet having either chronic constipation or diarrhea.

"There are only two ways to live your life. One is as though nothing is a miracle. The other is as though everything is a miracle."

-- *Albert Einstein*

The answer is right under my nose in *Pottenger's Cats*. Pottenger speaks of the cooked meat diet causing allergies, among other things, in cats. First deficient generation allergic cats produced second-generation kittens with greater incidence of allergies and by the third generation, the incidence was almost 100 percent.[53]

Pottenger stated in his study that the intestinal tracts of the allergic cats proved particularly remarkable at autopsy. Measurements of the length of the gastrointestinal tracts of several hundred normal and deficient adult cats were compared. The measurement started at the epiglottis and included the esophagus, the stomach, duodenum, jejunum and the colon to the rectum. In the average normal cat, the intestinal tract was approximately 48 inches long; in some of the allergic cats, the intestinal tracts measured as long as 72 to 80 inches. *Those elongated tracts lacked tissue tone and elasticity.*[54]

The digestive tract begins with the mouth. The cooked meat diet caused dental problems in the cats that progressively got worse from generation to generation. Adult cats placed on a cooked meat or pasteurized milk diet began to show unhealthy conditions in their mouths within three to six months. These cats first presented gingivitis followed by incrustation of salivary calculi that continued to increase whether the cat was maintained on a deficient diet or returned to an optimum diet.[55]

This is why tartar build-up often does not improve when a cat previously on a commercial food diet is put on a raw diet. A cleaning may be necessary to remove the tarter and if the cat remains on a raw diet that includes chunks of meat fed on a daily basis, the tartar should be minimal. An all-ground raw diet may not be enough to keep a cat's mouth completely healthy. They need the friction from chunks of raw meat for total dental health.

The second generation of cooked-meat fed cats showed irregular development of the skull cap and a narrowing of the malar and orbital arches. Most of the cats showed longer and narrower faces. In the second generation there was delay in loss of kitten teeth. Eruption of adult teeth was often accompanied by bleeding gums, runny noses and fevers. The adult teeth were usually smaller and more irregular in size. The degenerative changes became even more pronounced in the third generation.[56]

In Pottenger's study, two kittens born to a deficient mother were separated at approximately five weeks old. One kitten remained on a deficient diet. The other kitten was forced to forage for herself. The kitten on the deficient diet showed marked dental deformity. The foraging kitten showed the effects of her deficient history, but revealed major correction in the alignment of her teeth.[57] The ripping, cutting and tearing that a cat naturally engages in when eating his normal prey is critical to proper dental development. I believe ripping, tearing and cutting food is important throughout a cat's life.

If health problems such as dental issues and allergies began with Pottenger's cats on a cooked food diet and became progressively worse in the generations that followed, it stands to reason that kittens or young cats born to cats fed today's commercial food would have similar health issues. "Doctoring" the problem by adding more bulk to the diet or removing raw bone or bone meal and substituting a calcium product such as calcium citrate is only exacerbating the problem. Substituting a cooked, processed ingredient for a raw ingredient is not the answer.

I have to wonder if Pottenger would have seen such brilliant results had he used an animal other than cats in his study. Raw ingredients are so important to cats. Today's cats have the benefit of conventional medicine to nurse them through their degenerative illnesses. If a cat develops dental problems, teeth are pulled and sometimes in extreme cases all of the cat's teeth are pulled. If a cat has diarrhea, there are drugs for that, there are enemas and stool softeners for constipation. If someone wants to take a more natural approach, there are herbs like slippery elm, pumpkin to add bulk. There are antibiotics and steroids for everything else that goes wrong.

Too much bone or any form of calcium in a cat's diet *will* cause constipation! You should not feed a steady diet of chicken or turkey necks, backs or wings. There is too much bone in these cuts of poultry.

There is degenerative disease passing through generations. Years of cooked food is destroying the health of cats (and dogs and people and every other living being fed an improper diet). No matter how many new food formulations, vaccines, or drugs are developed, the health of cats is not going to improve until the root of the problem is addressed. Conventional medicine or practices is not the answer.

Both diarrhea and constipation can be resolved by proper use of homeopathy or other natural medicine, especially if it is in a young cat. I have had very few occurrences with constipation in my cats (all associated with another illness or confinement) and all resolved completely with homeopathy. Rarely do I have diarrhea in my cats and if I do it almost always resolves on its own in a day or two.

Here are some pictures of what I consider normal stools:

This is a perfectly-formed Tootsie Roll-type stool.

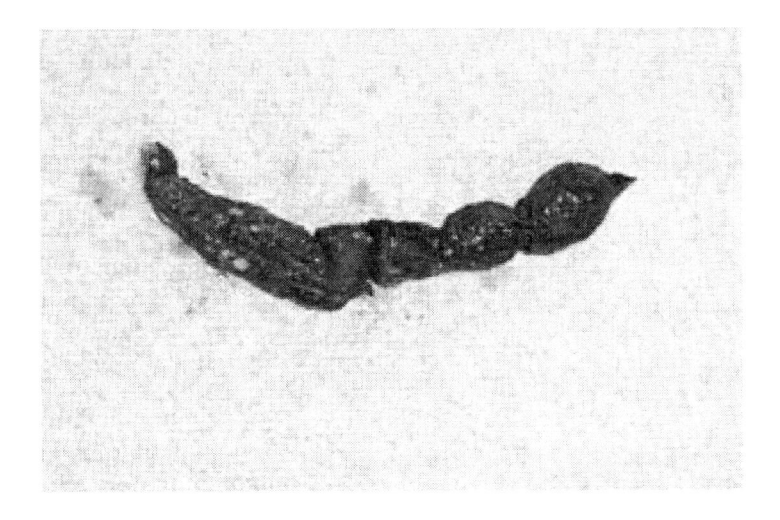

This is a stool that broke up some when being passed. The stool in this picture is perfectly fine. If your cat is consistently passing stool that consists of many small, round, dry balls, seek homeopathic help.

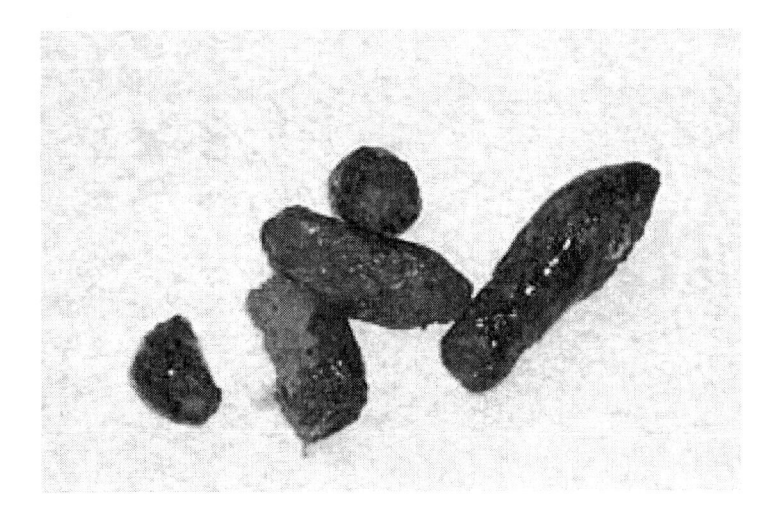

This is a stool that has been sitting out in the air. It is dried and multi-colored. This is what happens to my cats' stools when they have been exposed to air.

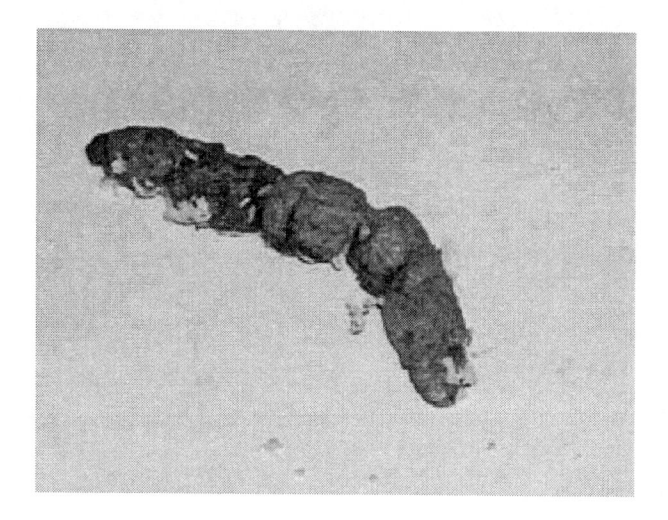

You may see occasional diarrhea, bloody, excessively smelly stools or mucus in your cat's stool. As long as it does not go on for more than a few days and there are no other symptoms such as lethargy or vomiting, I would not worry. If the meat you are feeding your cat is starting to turn, even slightly, it may cause your cat to have diarrhea. Diarrhea is a good thing, as long as it does not last for any length of time. Diarrhea is forcing toxins quickly out of the cat's digestive system. Suppressing the diarrhea is suppressing the cat's natural defense against toxic food. Remember, the diarrhea is there for a reason. You should try to discover and remove the *reason* for the diarrhea, not the diarrhea itself.

The calcium to phosphorus ratios of chicken or turkey legs (with the bone) or the whole animal (with the bone) are correct just the way they are. Mixing and matching pieces, for example grinding chicken necks and adding boneless chicken thigh may not be a huge problem, but it is better to use the leg (or whole animal). Then you can be sure the calcium to phosphorus ratio is correct. Chicken necks and backs have a high calcium to phosphorus ratio – there is too much bone and not enough muscle meat. Chicken necks and backs are fine to be fed on "prey night" (see Chapter 9), but not on a steady basis. Your cat may get constipated – it is too much bone. A constant diet of chicken wings may result in constipation as well.

Grinding

You are going to have to buy a grinder to feed this diet. You can buy an electric grinder or a hand crank model (which makes preparing the food a form of upper body exercise, and a lot more work). Information on where to purchase a grinder is shown on the shopping list included in this book.

I used the Maverick grinder for years. It recently died a peaceful death and I replaced it with the Tasin TS-108 grinder. The Maverick does a fine job, but you will need to cut the meat into small pieces to get it through the feed tube. I believe the Tasin grinder is superior because it has a larger feed tube, it will grind whole turkey thigh bone and the chopping plate is pie-shaped which results in a coarser grind. The Tasin grinder is also larger and sturdier than the Maverick grinder. If you are feeding more than a couple of cats, the Tasin grinder will probably work better for you.

Purchasing a grinder and the various supplements used for this diet is a significant investment. I believe you will find the enhanced health and well being of your cat far outweighs the initial investment and, in the long run, you may avoid costly visits to your veterinarian because you feed a raw diet.

With any grinder, use the cutting plate (the round thing that goes on the front of the grinder to hold the blade in place) with the largest holes.

If you want to grind turkey thighs with the bone, cut the meat off the bone, then smash the bone with a heavy cleaver to break it up. Do not try to put turkey bones through a Maverick or similar grinder before smashing them as it will damage the grinder. The Maverick grinder will not handle turkey drumstick bones, even if crushed. The Tasin grinder will handle turkey thigh bones whole, but it has a hard time with drumsticks.

The washable parts to both grinders can be run through the dishwasher, but they sometimes turn black or rust. It is better to wash them by hand and dry them thoroughly. I wrap the cutting blade and chopping plate in several pieces of paper towel to prevent them from rusting. If you live in a dry climate, you may not need to do this.

Commercially-prepared raw meat for pets

I usually do not advise purchasing meat ground by a commercial supplier of raw pet food. The only way I would buy meat ground by a butcher is if I can see what the butcher is grinding before it is ground and I am there to observe the process. Otherwise, you cannot be sure what is in the final product.

I believe the diet I detailed in this book is the optimum food you can feed your cat, however, I understand not everyone is willing to make the commitment to feeding this type of a diet. Any raw meat fed to your cat in addition to a commercial canned food product (I do not recommend any dry food product except perhaps Wysong's Archetype) is better than none. If you feed a small amount of raw meat in addition to canned food, you do not need to add any supplements. If the raw meat you feed in addition to commercial food is more than 15 percent of the diet, you should be sure is supplemented minimally with calcium to balance the phosphorus. One-third of a teaspoon of powdered eggshells or a tablespoon of human grade bone meal to one pound of meat is sufficient. If you feed meat with bone such as chicken necks, no supplemental calcium is necessary. If you feed raw meat to your cat several times a week and feed commercial canned food the rest of the time that is better than feeding 100 percent commercial food.

There is risk of contamination if the meat is ground elsewhere. The grinder used may not be as clean as you would keep your grinder. You do not know when the meat was ground or how long it was left out in the air. The moment that meat is ground it begins to oxidize. Whole poultry or rabbit parts will keep much longer than ground poultry or rabbit. Cats like their food extremely fresh. If it is starting to turn, even if you cannot smell it, your cat can and he may not eat the food.

Because ground meat loses its freshness so quickly, it is better to make small batches more frequently. Buying meat pre-ground may mean that you will have to buy a large quantity. My meat gets frozen whole, defrosted and prepared. I have enough cats so they go through a double recipe in a few days, thus I never have to freeze the ground meat with the supplements.

A good example of the potential problems associated with commercial grinding of meat occurred with the Winn Feline Foundation Study, *Role of Diet in the Health of the Feline Intestinal Tract and in Inflammatory Bowel Disease*. In the study, 22 adolescent cats were fed two different diets. One diet was a premium brand dry commercial kitten food, the other was whole ground rabbit obtained at a local rabbitry.

The rabbit was ground whole (including the fur and all the organs) and then frozen. The study went on for twelve months. Ten months into the study one of the cats on the rabbit diet died from dilated cardiomyopathy due to a severe taurine deficiency. Seventy percent of the remaining cats had heart muscle changes compatible with taurine deficiency.[58]

If you read between the lines of the study, you see where the problem arose. The researchers ascertained the raw ground rabbit contained the minimal requirement of taurine. They thought it possible that bacteria in the rabbit carcass or in the intestines of the cats broke down some of the taurine. Neither of these circumstances would be detrimental to diets containing excess levels of taurine, but would be detrimental if the diet was borderline deficient. In addition, vitamin E levels in the raw rabbit diet were low and this can cause the meat to lose taurine as it is processed and ground.[59]

The meat from grass-fed cattle is higher in vitamin E than those consuming grain, even higher than grain fed cattle fed supplemental vitamin E. In addition, the shelf life of grass-fed beef is longer than grain-fed beef.[60] It stands to reason a wild rabbit consuming grasses would have higher levels of vitamin E in its tissues than one consuming grain.

Grinding exposes more of the meat to oxygen causing it to oxygenate. Meat becomes oxidized after it is exposed to oxygen for 30 minutes. Vitamin E is an antioxidant and may help prevent or at least slow down oxidization.

The meat was ground by a commercial outfit (Rabbits were readily obtained from a rabbitry producing meat for human *and exotic animal consumption and were of comparatively low cost)*.[61] Bacteria would have been present since they ground the whole rabbit including the digestive organs. A cat consuming an adult rabbit would most likely not eat the stomach and intestines and if the stomach and intestines are consumed, it is while the animal is still fresh and whole, not after it has been ground and frozen. There also may have been bacteria present from the grinding process. Vitamin E levels were low because the meat was ground and frozen. Freezing or storage for any length of time can destroy vitamin E.

Wild cats in some parts of the world exist almost entirely on rabbit.[62] I believe it was including ground digestive organs in the mix and freezing the meat ground that destroyed the taurine. Changing the physical structure of a cat's food (grinding) and long-term storage can be detrimental to the cat.

The researchers looked at what a cat might eat in developing what they called a "gold standard diet" but they ignored *how* a cat eats. Their food is consumed fresh and it is eaten whole. It is so very important to look at the whole picture, not just one part of it.

I have cats weaned on rabbit that have gone on to reproduce normally. They have no signs of taurine deficiency. The rabbit I feed to my cats is not all ground, much of it is chunked and I usually do not grind the meat and then freeze it. I freeze whole rabbits, defrost, grind and feed.

If you are feeding one or two cats, you will need to freeze your prepared food. Try to make the time to make single batches once or twice a week instead of making many batches at a time and freezing them. Unless you are absolutely pressed for time, do not grind a huge quantity of meat, mix in the supplements and freeze it any length of time. Fresh is best.

If you feel you need to grind a large portion of meat and freeze it – add additional vitamin E to help prevent further oxidization and taurine prior to feeding it. If you are defrosting serving sized packages for one cat, you should be sure your cat is getting approximately 500 mg taurine on a daily basis. You probably do not need to add additional vitamin E or taurine if you are only freezing your meat for a week or two.

It is never ideal to freeze meat, thaw it, grind it and refreeze it, but I know in some instances this is necessary. Try to avoid doing this as much as possible. Let the meat defrost in your refrigerator.

When you are ready to grind your meat, it is easier to work with if you partially freeze it. The skin comes off the chicken easier and it is less difficult to cut the meat off the bone. I found that a good pair of poultry or kitchen shears is better for cutting poultry (or rabbit) than a knife. Cut the meat off the bone, chunk it and then grind the bone and the organ meat. If your cat is new to raw food it will take him time to learn to manage chunks of food. Make the chunks quite small until he gets used to the texture of the food. If he leaves the chunks and eats only the ground, put the chunks away for the next meal and offer only chunks. If necessary, cut them up smaller and gradually increase the size until your cat eats them without hesitation.

Dental health

Do not grind all of the meat! Cats do not eat ground food in the wild and you should not feed meat that is completely ground. It is the texture of the chunks of meat against the teeth and gums that does the cleaning. Unlike dogs, small cats do not gnaw on bones. While a larger cat may consume animals with large bones, our smaller cats hunt small prey animals. The bones of a small rodent or bird are quite fragile. It is not the bones of the prey that keep a wild cat's teeth clean and gums healthy — it is the abrasion of muscle meat against the teeth and gums that does the cleaning. When fed a proper diet (raw meat) a cat's mouth remains acidic. An acidic mouth inhibits bacteria growth. A cat eating a cereal-based diet (or even a raw diet that contains vegetables or grains) will lean more towards the alkaline side. A diet consisting entirely of raw ground meat is probably not enough to keep a cat's mouth healthy — you need those chunks for optimum dental health.

While it is perfectly acceptable to feed chicken necks or wings to your cats, I choose not to. Cats will avoid chewing on bones that are too hard to avoid breaking their teeth. Conventional sized chicken bones are larger and harder than small rodent or bird bones. My largest cat, Rooney, runs close to 15 pounds. He can handle full-sized chicken bones. The rest of my cats are considerably smaller. I rely on chunks of meat and sometimes cut-up Cornish Game Hens to keep their teeth and gums healthy.

Chicken or turkey necks

Use chicken necks as natural toothbrushes, not as a regular part of your cat's diet. The calcium to phosphorus ratio of chicken or turkey necks is not correct for long-term feeding. There is not enough meat on the bone of chicken or turkey necks. If you feed chicken necks too frequently, you risk your cat getting constipated. Turkey necks are too large for most cats to handle. If you can source Cornish Game Hen necks, those are wonderful for cats.

The beauty of raw meat

Your cat, as an obligate carnivore needs meat to thrive and it should be raw. Cats do not hunt their prey with a frying pan on their backs. I have never caught my cats playing with matches or attempting to cook their food. Believe me, they are smart enough to cook their food if they really want to. They do want their food served warm. They eat their prey warm. Put a serving in a cheap plastic bag and place it in a bath of warm water for fifteen minutes or so. That should warm it sufficiently. Do not microwave it! Microwaving changes the chemical structure of the protein and decreases its nutritional value.[63] Because you are working with a number of fragile supplements (vitamin E and salmon oil), you do not want to risk lowering the nutritional value of the food you work so hard to prepare.

"Microwave ovens are generally safe ... But they can alter the chemistry of protein foods cooked in them for long periods of time."
Andrew Weil, M.D.

The vitamins and minerals in meat are what a cat needs to stay healthy. For example, the supplement Co-enzyme Q-10 has been used to help cats with gum and heart disease. Co-enzyme Q-10 is naturally resident in meat, particularly the heart. If you are feeding a diet of raw meat, including heart, your cat is getting natural Co-enzyme Q-10.

Another supplement is L-Lysine that is used by many people to help cats with herpes virus (a common feline upper respiratory virus). L-Lysine is naturally occurring in raw meat.

While it may seem extremely time consuming at first, once you get the process down, you will be able to make up a batch of food in under an hour including cleanup. You will find time saving tips in a later chapter. I do not think an hour or two a week is a lot to invest into making excellent food for your cat.

Chapter 6 - Amino Acids

There are many nutrients cats must have in their diets, like the amino acids taurine and arginine, which can only be obtained from meat.

Taurine

Most people know a cat needs a high amount of taurine in his diet. This need was discovered quite by accident when cats started to show taurine deficiencies while fed commercial cat food containing the then recommend levels of 400 mg/kg of food.

The recommend levels of taurine were raised to the current levels of 1,000 mg/kg in dry food and 2,000 – 2,500 mg/kg in canned food. Cats fed canned foods require a higher quantity of taurine than those fed dry foods because of alterations in the bioavailability of taurine attributed to the effects of processing. However, despite the routine supplementation of commercial feline diets with taurine, cats continue to be diagnosed with taurine deficiency.[64] Requirements for taurine are influenced by dietary factors. For example, a cat consuming a high fiber diet would need more dietary taurine.

Cats have a limited ability to synthesize taurine from methionine and cysteine, therefore they need a reliable supply of taurine in their diet. Taurine is an extremely important amino acid involved in a large number of metabolic processes. It is important for visual pathways, the brain and nervous system, cardiac function and normal bile salt formation. Taurine is also important for proper reproduction and fetal development as well as immune function. It takes a prolonged period (five months to two years) for clinical signs of taurine deficiency to occur.[65]

I highly recommend doing the legwork and sourcing raw heart to use to make your cat food instead of using taurine supplement. Heart is rich in taurine and other essential nutrients. Remember, heart is not just taurine. As you will see from in Table 5, heart is a rich source of niacin and potassium, both important to cats.

Table 5 - An analysis of 200 grams of raw chicken heart

Nutrient	Total
Calories	306
Pro (g)	31.2
Fat (g)	18.6
Carb (g)	1.4

Nutrient	Total
Fiber (g)	0
Cal (mg)	24
Iron (mg)	12
Na (mg)	148
Pot (mg)	352
Phos (mg)	354
Ash (g)	1.8
vitA (IU)	60
vitC (mg)	6.4
Thia (mg)	0.3
Ribo (mg)	1.46
Nia (mg)	9.76
H2O %	73.6
satF (g)	5.32
monoF (g)	4.74
polyF (g)	5.42
Chol (mg)	272

Analysis completed using the Nutritional Analysis Tool 2.0 **http://www.nat.uiuc.edu**

You may wonder why there is a half a pound of heart in the recipe. Of course the heart of the prey of a small cat is not going to amount to 20 percent of the entire weight of the animal, however, mice are quite high in taurine. One thousand grams of mouse carcass has 7,000 mg taurine on a dry matter basis.[66] I know that sounds like a lot of taurine, but before you start dumping supplemental taurine into your cat's food, if you hydrate the mouse by 70 percent it comes out to about 2,100 mg per 1,000 grams.

I have been unable to locate information on the amount of taurine in raw chicken heart. You will note in Table 6, the taurine in pig heart is significantly higher than that in pork muscle meat. This is intended as an example, I do not recommend feeding pork. Table 6 was part of a study of a Chinese human diet and I believe the values are for cooked meat. The values for raw meat are considerably higher. Taurine is not recognized as an essential amino acid for adult humans so nutritional databases do not list taurine in their amino acid profiles. You will note from the table below that there is more taurine in chicken leg than in chicken breast.

Table 6 - Taurine Content in Various Foods

Taurine content of meats, poultry and aquatic products in China (mg/100g edible portion)

Food	Taurine conc.	Food	Taurine conc.
Conch	850	Hairtail fish	56
Inkfish	672	Yellow croaker	88
Blood clam	617	Eel	91
Clam	496	Chicken leg	378
Shellfish	332	Chicken breast	26
Crab	278	Pork	118
Prawn	143	Pig heart	200
Sole	256	Pig kidney	120
Crucial carp	205	Pig liver	42
Silver carp	90	Beef	64

Table from Zhao Xi-he, *Dietary Protein, Amino Acids and Their Relation to Health*, Asia Pacific J Clin Nutr (1994), 3, 131-134.

Taurine is present in most raw meat and eggs. While taurine is available in muscle meat, it is most abundant in the heart and brain. It is present only in trace amounts in plants. Taurine does occur in red algae, but not in brown or green algae. Taurine is also present in high levels in insects.

For years I fed a raw meat diet to my cats and did not supplement with taurine, nor did I add heart. It is hard to say whether the improved immune function I see in my cats is due to the additional taurine they are now getting or that they have simply become healthier the longer they have been on raw and cared for holistically. It is most likely a combination of both.

Do the legwork, find raw heart (chicken if you are using chicken, turkey, or rabbit; and beef if you are feeding beef) and use it in your cat food. Do not use supplemental taurine unless you absolutely have to. Ethnic stores, such as Chinese and Mexican grocery stores, often have chicken hearts. Butchers may be able to source them. I purchase 20 pounds of chicken hearts and 10 pounds of chicken liver at a time. I bag up 200 grams of chicken heart and 100 grams of chicken liver for a double recipe and store them in zipper freezer bags and freeze them.

Freeze your heart and liver whole, not ground. This is an instance where you may have to freeze, thaw, and refreeze because most people have to buy their heart and liver in bulk in order to have a reliable supply. When adding the chicken heart and liver to your meat, do not throw out the excess blood.

If you can source whole chickens or rabbits, use the heads! There is a reason why a cat usually eats his prey head first.[67][68]

If you are using raw heart and are still concerned about taurine in your cat's diet, there is no problem with adding additional powdered taurine to the recipe.

Mixing Proteins

People ask about using beef heart with chicken or visa versa. I do not believe that is a good idea. First of all, it is possible to source both chicken and beef heart, therefore, if you are using chicken, you should use chicken heart; if you are using beef, use beef heart. It makes more sense to keep the meat you are feeding your cat from the same species of animal. With a regular recipe using chicken, you are feeding your cat protein from three different sources, chicken – which includes muscle meat, bone, heart and liver, egg and salmon oil. If you make the same recipe using chicken muscle meat, chicken liver, beef heart and egg – that is four different protein sources. I believe that is overloading a cat's digestive system. I cannot offer much more of a reason for not mixing species other than it does not make sense and in some cats it causes digestive upset. It may not cause problems right away, but over time, you may see symptoms similar to inflammatory bowel disease in your cat. I often wonder if the multiple protein sources included in commercial food may be one cause of feline inflammatory bowel disease. This would explain why veterinarians often suggest a commercial food containing a single protein source. You are trying to replicate a cat's natural diet. Mixing species is counter to what a cat would eat in his wild state.

Arginine

Arginine is perhaps more important to the cat than taurine. Feeding foods devoid of arginine can result in hyperammonemia (a metabolic disorder marked by elevated concentrations of ammonia or ammonium ions in blood) in less than one hour. If a cat eats an arginine-deficient meal, the highly active protein catabolic enzymes in its liver produce ammonia. Without arginine, the urea cycle cannot convert ammonia to urea and ammonia toxicity occurs. Urea cycle enzymes are nonadaptive in cats, whereas in omnivores the activity of these enzymes changes in response to changing dietary protein levels. The urea cycle cleans up during protein metabolism and disposes of nitrogen wastes via the liver and kidneys.

Cats have lost flexibility in protein metabolism seen in other animal species that eat foods with a more varied protein content. Because a cat's natural diet *has always been reliably high in protein*, there was little evolutionary drive toward adaptive metabolic enzyme systems.[69]

As with taurine, arginine is readily available in meat and eggs.

Miscellaneous amino acids

Methionine and cystine are required in higher amounts in cats than most other species. Both are present in high amounts in meat and eggs.

Tyrosine is an amino acid that is not essential for other species, but is considered to be conditionally essential for cats. This amino acid plays an important role in the synthesis and homeostatis of melanin, which is found in black hair and skin pigment. Tyrosine is synthesized from phenylalanine, an amino acid contained in many proteins. Tyrosine deficiency is most commonly observed in black cats whose hair becomes reddish-brown. Tyrosine is readily available in animal-source proteins.[70] This explains why my black cats have always been very rich black in color and have never rusted. I always thought "rusting" was due to some chemical in commercial cat food.

Carnitine is an amino-group containing, vitamin-like substance found in high concentrations in mammalian heart and skeletal muscle. The AAFCO may eventually determine it to be an essential amino acid. Cats can synthesize carnitine from lysine and methionine (both found in meat). In humans, a carnitine deficiency causes hepatic lipid accumulation and liver dysfunction. A similar connection is being investigated in cats. Also, carnitine increases lean muscle mass and enhances weight loss in obese cats.[71]

A diet high in raw animal flesh provides all of the amino acids a cat needs.

Chapter 7 - Fats and Fatty Acids

Cats have the *ability* to digest and use high levels of dietary fat from animal tissues. While they have the ability to digest and use high levels of fat and they like the taste of fat, their natural prey is *low* in fat. Cats may be able to the to "tolerate" and "digest" cardboard, but is it good for them?

Keep the amount of fat you feed your cat low and high in quality. If you can source free-range chickens, you are way ahead of the game. If I feed conventionally raised chicken to my cats, I remove the skin. Yes, skin contains a high amount of vitamin D, but so do liver and egg yolks. The problem with the fat of a conventionally raised chicken or cow is that it throws off the omega 6 to omega 3 fatty acid ratios. Chicken fat is high in the omega 6 fatty acid, arachidonic acid (AA), which cats need in their diets, however, AA is also present in muscle and organ meat and eggs. Using the chicken skin makes the entire meal too high in omega 6 fatty acids. In general, omega 6 fatty acids are pro-inflammatory and omega 3 fatty acids are anti-inflammatory. Any food that causes inflammatory conditions should not be fed in excess, especially if your cat is at all prone to any inflammatory condition such as allergies or IBD.

Many animals, such as dogs, can synthesize arachidonic acid from linoleic acid (LA). Arachidonic acid is abundant in animal tissues, particularly organ meats and neural tissues (nerve tissues like the brain, eyes [optic nerves and retina] and spinal cord). Plants do not contain arachidonic acid.

The omega 3 fatty acids, eicosapentaenoic acid (EPA) and docosahexaenoic acid (DHA), are not considered by the AAFCO to be essential to cats or dogs, however, they are extremely beneficial as they are anti-inflammatory. Because of their anti-inflammatory action, omega 3 fatty acids have become vogue and some high-end pet food brands have started to add them to their pet food. Unfortunately, omega 3 fatty acids in most brands of pet food will be from plant sources such as borage or flax oils. Cats are unable to convert omega fatty acids from plant sources. A reliable supplemental source of EPA and DHA for cats is salmon oil in capsules. In their natural prey, EPA is present in the tissues and DHA is present in the neural tissues.

Researchers discovered if they supplement chicken feed with fish oils, the chickens were less prone to the coccidia (a single celled organism that infects the intestine and can effect many types of mammals and birds) .[72] Cats, especially those living in a multi-cat environment, can contract coccidia as it is spread through feces and is difficult to remove from the environment. Perhaps if cats were fed a bioavailable form of omega 3 fatty acids like salmon oil they would be less prone to coccidia. Even though they are out chasing my flock of free-range chickens and they occasionally catch and consume birds, my cats and kittens remain free from coccidia.

Here is a listing of natural sources for various omega fatty acids:

Linoleic Acid (LA) is an omega 6 fatty acid found in processed foods like margarine and vegetable oils, as well as in evening primrose oil, grape seed oil, flax seed oil and other vegetable oils. LA may be converted to GLA and AA in humans and healthy dogs.

Alpha Linolenic Acid (often referred to as just Linolenic Acid) (ALA) is an omega 3 fatty acid found in flax oil and black currant oil. Humans and healthy dogs convert some ALA to EPA and DHA.

Gamma Linolenic Acid (GLA) is an omega 6 fatty acid found in borage, black currant and evening primrose oils. Healthy humans and healthy dogs can convert LA to GLA.

Eicosapentaenoic Acid and Docosahexaenoic Acid (EPA and DHA) are both omega 3 fatty acids found in fatty fish such as salmon, mackerel, tuna and sardines.

Arachidonic Acid (AA) is an omega 6 fatty acid found in meat, eggs and some shellfish.

You will note that LA, ALA and GLA are all found in plant sources. EPA, DHA and AA, all essential for cats, are from animal sources. That makes sense since cats naturally eat animals not plants. The omega fatty acids you feed your cats should come from animal sources, not plants.

EPA would be available to the cat in the tissues of the prey animals it consumed as long as these prey animals were consuming their natural diet (grass, plants and seeds). DHA is present in the neural tissues of the prey. Unless you are feeding whole prey animals (including the head) from animals who are consuming their natural food, a bioavailable form of EPA and DHA should be in the food you feed to your cats.

Fish who feed on marine plants, especially fatty fish like salmon, anchovies, sardines and mackerel contain both EPA and DHA in their tissues. While some brands of cod liver oil may contain omega 3 fatty acids, it is not advisable to use cod liver oil as a source of omega 3 fatty acids because cod liver oil is extremely high in vitamins A and D.

There is controversy as to whether farmed salmon contains sufficient levels of EPA and DHA in their tissues. Wild salmon convert the LNA in marine plants into EPA and DHA. Cows that eat grass have EPA in their tissues while those fed grain do not. Farmed salmon are fed grain, not marine plants. To counter this, many "salmon" oil capsules contain other fatty fish besides salmon to bring up the EPA and DHA levels. That is perfectly fine, but if you can source wild salmon oil, use it.

Do not be misled into using vegetable oils like flax or safflower oil to provide essential fatty acids to your cat. Healthy dogs appear to be able to convert the essential fatty acid, ALA, contained in flax oil to EPA and DHA, but remember dogs are a bit more flexible in their digestion abilities; they are able to get some of their nutrition from plant sources. Healthy dogs can convert LA (which is contained in safflower oil) to AA, cats cannot.

> *"We must be the change we wish to see in the world."*
> *-- Mahatma Gandhi*

Do not mess with Mother Nature. Mice eat seeds and grass and convert the omega 3 fatty acids in the seeds and grass into EPA and DHA. Cats eat the mice and obtain AA, EPA and DHA from the tissues of the mouse. Since you cannot feed tasty field mice to your cats, use lean, raw meat for the AA and salmon oil for the EPA and DHA.

If a required nutrient can be derived from an animal source, then that is what you should feed. Do not rely on non-animal ingredients to provide nutrition for your cat. If you are going to put the effort into feeding your cat a raw diet, then you should make it as species-appropriate as possible.

Chapter 8 - Organ Meat

I have already addressed heart in a previous chapter. The other organ you will need to feed your cat on nearly a daily basis in minimal amounts is raw liver. Liver is a rich source of vitamin A and other nutrients. See Table 7 for an analysis of chicken liver.

Table 7 - An analysis of 100 grams of raw chicken liver

Nutrient	Total
Calories	125
Pro (g)	18
Fat (g)	3.9
Carb (g)	3.4
Fiber (g)	0
Cal (mg)	11
Iron (mg)	8.6
Na (mg)	79
Pot (mg)	228
Phos (mg)	272
Ash (g)	1.2
vitA (IU)	20549
vitC (mg)	33.8
Thia (mg)	0.14
Ribo (mg)	1.96
Nia (mg)	9.25
H2O percent	73.6
satF (g)	1.3
monoF (g)	0.95
polyF (g)	0.64
Chol (mg)	439

Analysis completed using the Nutritional Analysis Tool 2.0 **http://www.nat.uiuc.edu**

There have been instances of vitamin A overdose in cats, therefore, I caution against feeding much more than 100 grams of liver per week. There was a study conducted wherein cats were fed a diet containing 150 to 300 times the vitamin A requirement for a period of three to four years with no ill effects.[73] In light of that study I am not too concerned with a vitamin A overdose in my cats.

A cat's natural prey is high in vitamin A. 1,000 grams of mouse carcass has 20,000 to 30,000 IU vitamin A.[74]

Table 8 – An Analysis of vitamin A in a sample recipe using chicken

Food	Vitamin A (IU)
2 large raw chicken yolks	645.74
100 grams raw chicken liver	20,549[1]
200 grams raw chicken heart	60
700 grams raw chicken thigh (no skin)	455
1000 grams of excellent cat food	21,709.74 IU

Analysis completed using the Nutritional Analysis Tool 2.0 **http://www.nat.uiuc.edu**

Given the levels of vitamin A in various prey species, I do not think 21,709.74 IU of vitamin A is excessive. Cats eat animals that have livers. I see no reason why cats should not receive a small amount of liver every day. One hundred grams of chicken liver (the amount used in the recipe) amounts to about two large chicken livers. Vitamin A is quite important for immune function and skin health. Given the poor immune systems of cats today as well as the prevalence of skin disease in cats, perhaps the AAFCO-recommended 5,000 IU per kg of food is too low. It may keep a cat alive, but most of us want to do more than keep our cats alive. We want them to thrive. The AAFCO lists a maximum of vitamin A as 750,000 IU per kg of food. We are not even close to that.

Interestingly, taurine and zinc, both found in animal foods, provide protection from excess vitamin A – a vitamin found only in animal foods.

Organic animals are not given routine drugs or fed animal by-products, therefore, it is better to use organic organ meat if you can source it. If you feed organic meat and organ meat, there is less chance of drug or toxin build up in the tissues.

Chicken gizzards are perfectly fine to feed to cats, although some cats do not like them. If you use them in a recipe they are considered muscle meat. If included in a recipe using meat with bone, you will need to adjust the calcium levels. If you are math challenged (like me) this can be difficult. Use chicken gizzards on prey night. They provide excellent chewing exercise.

Another fat soluble vitamin that cats should receive in their food is vitamin D. Unlike some animals, cats cannot synthesize vitamin D from the sun because they have insufficient 7-dehydrocholestrol in their skin to meet their metabolic need for vitamin D photosynthesis.[75] The researchers who conducted the study

---

[1] Beef liver is considerably higher in vitamin A – 100 grams contains 35,346 IU.

quoted in the previous footnote ascertained that analysis of wild caught prey of cats indicated that these animals could supply adequate vitamin D to meet the requirement of growing kittens.[76]

Marine fish and fish oils are the richest natural sources of vitamin D in foodstuffs *but they may pose a risk for toxicity.* Other sources of vitamin D include fresh water fish and eggs (especially yolks). Beef, liver and dairy products contain smaller amounts of vitamin D. Animal fat also contains vitamin D.

As cats have existed for millions of years as a species without resorting to deep-sea fishing, I would have to assume a diet consisting of raw meat, including liver will provide sufficient vitamin D.

Chapter 9 - Feeding Prey Animals – "Prey Night"

The absolute ideal food you can feed to your cat is small prey animals such as naturally raised mice or other small rodents, insects and small birds. Keep in mind that in order to be absolutely perfect packages of nutrition for your cat, these animals must be fed their natural diet, not commercial food. This is virtually impossible for most people. I have raised and fed mice in the past. Keeping mice is a smelly business. They stink to high heaven!

Frozen prey animals are an option. Be absolutely certain they are from a reliable source. Remember that mice are often used as laboratory animals. Who knows what these laboratory mice are fed, injected or medicated with? I also worry about the chemicals used in euthanizing the mice.

If you have the facilities to raise mice, then by all means do so. Feed your mice a species-appropriate diet of seeds and grasses. Do not feed commercial mouse food — it has more chemicals in it than conventional cat food.

The other difficulty with feeding mice is that many cats do not recognize them as "food." Unless they are taught to kill and eat mice at an early age, they do not know what to do with a small furry creature besides torture it to death.

People ask how I "taught" my cats to eat mice. I started with a pregnant cat. Pregnant and nursing cats will eat almost anything that does not eat them first. I offered Trompe (who was almost due to deliver kittens), a dead mouse I had cut in half. She tried it and ate it. I then put her in a cage and offered her a live mouse. She figured out very quickly how to efficiently kill and eat it. Several of my other cats learned how to kill and eat mice by observing Trompe.

Wiley was a very efficient killer and eater of mice. I considered renting him out as a mouse exterminator. I am sure he would have had a ball. He is probably catching and eating his share of tasty field mice in Heaven.

Even though you should always have chunks in the mixture you feed your cats, providing your cat with the "whole prey" experience is important. Alternatives to feeding live or frozen prey animals are Cornish Game Hens either cut up or whole, squab, quail, chunks of stew beef or lamb, chicken necks, or chicken wings. Feed these pseudo-prey animals as a meal two or three times a week.

Chapter 10 - Variety

There has been some criticism about lack of variety in this type of diet. I do not feed different supplements on different days. I feed organ meat, including liver, just about every day. In their wild state, cats eat perfect packages of nutrition. Their mice, rabbits and other prey all have livers, hearts, gall bladders and spleens. They also have muscle meat, bone and hide. I try to replicate that diet. My cats get variety in the types of meat they eat. They eat predominantly rabbit and chicken, with other types of meat (such as beef, lamb and venison) thrown in for good measure. Sometimes they get crickets, they catch flies, moths and other bugs. I am confident my cats are getting as much variety in their diet as a wild cat would.

I do not want to worry about what day my cats got liver, what day they got salmon oil, or what day they got vitamin E. They get these ingredients in every meal, except for prey nights when they get chunks of meat or prey animals. Perfect packages of nutrition is what we strive for here at Blakkatz, not balance over time. I live in the moment and I make the best of what I feed my cats in every meal. Why leave for tomorrow what you can do today?

There are many cats that refuse to eat certain types of meat and some who can only tolerate certain types of meat. The raw egg yolks and vitamin B complex help round out the diet and make up for any deficiencies. Rooney refuses to eat anything other than poultry and when offered, fish. He wouldn't eat rabbit, beef, or lamb. I have seen no signs of deficiency in Rooney that could be attributed to a diet of mostly poultry. Rooney is my resident poultry aficionado.

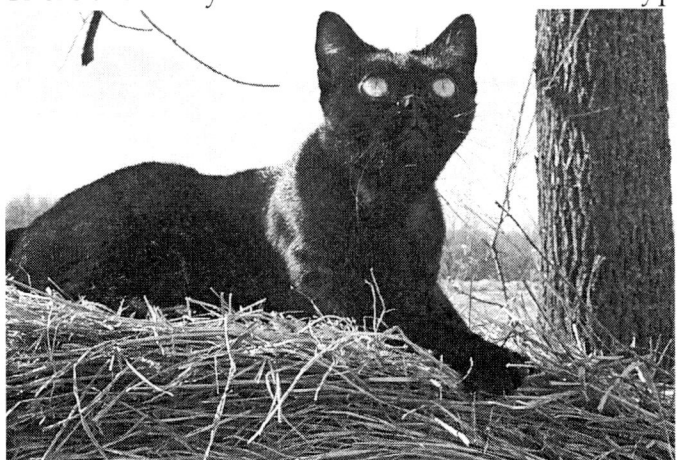

Chapter 11 - Carbohydrates and Fiber

I do not advocate feeding anything to a cat that contains carbohydrates (such as grains or vegetables). While there is the possibility that a cat may be able to derive some nutritional benefits from plants, that is not how they are designed by nature to eat. Cats eat animals that eat plants. Animals that eat plants are designed very differently than those that eat animals. Cats are obligate carnivores. They do not, under normal conditions, eat plants. I know some cats will steal and eat vegetables from their caregiver's plate. I believe this is for several reasons. Cats who have been on a commercial food diet for any length of time may continue to crave carbohydrates. Also, stealing is very feline. Mine steal food quite frequently. Put a plate of vegetables and a plate of raw meat in front of your cat and see which one he'll eat. I will put money on the meat plate. My cats who have been weaned on raw, like Tangle shown in the photograph, would not be caught dead eating vegetables!

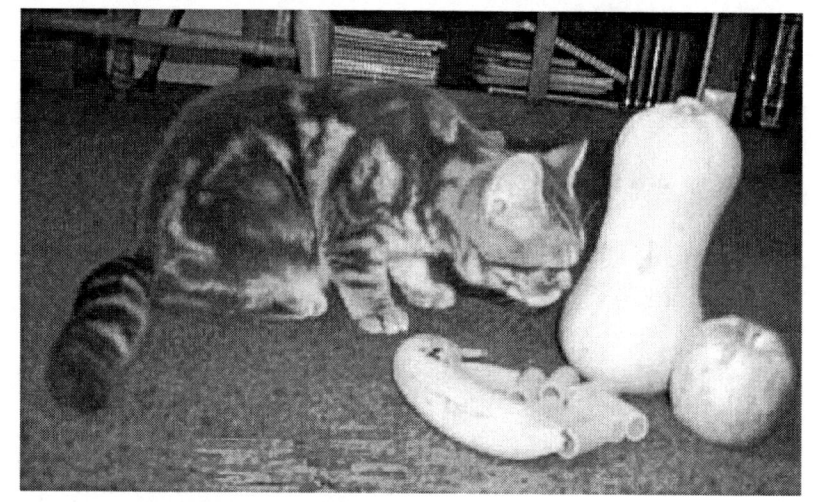

Along with sharp claws, cats have powerful jaws and pointed, elongated, canine teeth to spear and tear flesh. They do not have molars which grazing animals need for grinding their food. In fact cats do not have any flat teeth in their mouth. Their jaws have limited ability to move from side to side to grind food. Unlike plants and grains, flesh does not need to be chewed in the mouth to predigest it, rather it is digested in the stomach. Cats lack salivary amylase used to initiate digestion of plants.

Cats can hardly chew at all. They use their "carnassial" (a tooth adapted for tearing apart flesh, especially one of the last upper premolar or first lower molar teeth in carnivorous mammals) teeth like shears to cut their food into manageable pieces. When my cats vomit even hours after eating, the food comes back up pretty much the way it went in. They will often swallow a mouse whole.

The intestines of cats are markedly shorter than that of omnivores or herbivores. A cat's small intestinal length compared to its body length is 4:1, a rabbit's is

10:1, a pig 14:1.[77] The small intestine of cats is not adaptive to varying levels of dietary carbohydrates. Cats do not waste energy or nitrogen by turning over carriers or enzyme systems of little value because free sugars and complex carbohydrates would normally make up a negligible percentage of their food.[78] For example, a rat carcass is comprised of 1.2 percent carbohydrates and 0.55 percent fiber.[79] One hundred grams of mouse carcass consists of 1.7 percent crude fiber on a dry matter basis.[80]

The feline liver has several unique features that are evident in energy metabolism. In omnivores the enzymes hexokinase and glucokinase are responsible for the conversion of glucose to energy. Cats have very low liver glucokinase activity and a limited ability to metabolize large amounts of simple carbohydrates because their natural diet is high in protein and low in carbohydrates. Low glucokinase activity, though practical in a species consuming little carbohydrates, limits the cat's ability to metabolize large amounts of carbohydrates.[81]

Although cats are physiologically deficient in carbohydrate metabolism, pet food manufacturers claim that cats "tolerate" dry food that contains 40% or more dietary carbohydrates. Grains were added to commercial pet food as cheap filler. Grain, especially grain by-product, is less expensive than meat. High-gluten formations (mostly wheat) are necessary to provide product shape and rigidity.[82] While the energy and protein levels of commercial cat food look proper on paper, if cats cannot digest plant material or easily convert carbohydrates to energy, how are they going to derive proper nourishment from commercial cat food?

A wild cat expends a tremendous amount of energy in order to survive and they do not consume carbohydrates.

Cats have a *nonfunctioning* cecum and a short colon. The cecum is a blind-ending pouch near the beginning of the large intestine that provides additional space for digestion in herbivores. In some plant-eating animals, such as cows, the cecum contains special bacteria that aid in the digestion of cellulose. These anatomic features limit the cat's capability to use poorly digestible starches and fiber by microbial fermentation in the large bowel.[83] Fermentation of fiber by colonic bacteria may yield short chain fatty acids that are an important energy source for cattle and horses (short chain fatty acids can supply up to 75 percent of daily energy requirements in cows and horses). They provide less than 5 percent of the energy needs of dogs and cats because of the short intestinal tract and relatively fast transit time in those species.[84]

Some pet food manufacturers add ingredients such as sodium bentonite, powdered cellulose, beet pulp, tomato (or any other) pomace and ground peanut shells to slow intestinal transit time. Otherwise their food would result in extremely soft and frequent stools, something no cat guardian wants. Slowing intestinal transit time can be dangerous because cats need to be able to expel food from their system if it is toxic in some manner. That is why cats vomit so easily. It is a safeguard against poisoning from raw meat.

Remember, cats are not humans, horses, or cows. Cats are obligate carnivores and must eat meat to survive. They are virtually unable to digest plant material. Vegetables and grains go right through them with the cat deriving little nutritional benefit.

Feeding vegetables and grains to a cat results in big, smelly, nasty stools! Not too long ago, as an experiment, I added freshly grown wheat grass to my cats' food in place of their usual fiber (psyllium husk powder). Instead of nicely formed Tootsie Roll stools they started passing giant, soft, smelly stools. I turned my cats into carnivorous cows! It took several weeks to get their stools back to normal after I took the grass out of their food.

As I am walking out in the fields these days I wonder about picking a bunch of wild grass, taking it home, cooking it to death, running it through a food processor and then adding a very small amount of the cooked, processed mixture to my cats' food. Then I think, get real – that is too much work! It may replicate, to some extent, what a mouse would have in its stomach, but you cannot account for the actual digestive process of the mouse by cooking and processing.

While feeding a cat a small amount of carbohydrates may do no harm, it is fiber that you really want to be sure you are getting into your cat. While some cats may have no difficulty passing stools on a diet that contains no fiber, many will have uncomfortably hard stools. Vegetables provide some fiber, but they also provide carbohydrates. For example, Table 9 provides a break down of a few vegetables showing the carbohydrates and fiber they add to a diet.

Table 9 – a Breakdown of Fiber and Carbohydrates in Popular Vegetables

Vegetable (100 grams)	Carbohydrates (grams)	Fiber
Broccoli	5.06	2.9
Summer Squash	4.31	1.4
Carrots	10.48	3.3
Pumpkin, canned	8.08	2.9

Analysis completed using the Nutritional Analysis Tool 2.0 **http://www.nat.uiuc.edu**

Assuming you will want seven grams of fiber in a recipe of 1,000 grams of meat (the approximate amount of fiber in 1,000 grams of mouse carcass[85]), you will need to add quite a bit of vegetable to reach 7 grams of fiber. For example, you will need to add approximately 300 grams of broccoli to reach 7 grams of fiber. Many cats will object to that much vegetable matter in their food.

Most vegetables are not high in fiber. You could add cooked beans, but you will probably cause flatulence in your cat.

Vegetables are alkaline and meat is acidic. A cat's system should be acidic (a human's should be more alkaline). An alkaline or less acidic urine is thought to be a contributing factor to Feline Urological Syndrome (or Feline Lower Urinary Tract Disease). Cats on high meat diets naturally have acidic urine. The average urinary pH of a cat fed a normal diet is approximately 6.3.[86]

The other problem with feeding alkaline foods instead of acidic foods to cats is dental disease – which is quite common in cats these days. A cat's mouth should be acidic; feeding an alkaline food could make the mouth less acidic. In general, bacteria survive better in an alkaline pH than an acid pH.

I remember the days when I boiled huge soup pots of mixed vegetables. I cooked the vegetables to death then drained the vegetables reserving the cooking liquid. In the cooking liquid I cooked brown rice or some other whole grain. While the grains were cooking, I ran the vegetables through the food processor until they were baby food consistency. Once the grains were well cooked I ran those through the food processor as well. I mixed the grains and vegetables together into a sticky, gooey mess and froze it in zip lock bags. I added the grain/vegetable mixture to meat, sometimes as much as 40 percent of the mixture was grain/vegetable.

Cats have evolved as predators. They have been so successful as predators that they have never had to develop the ability to digest anything other than prey animals. Sure, they may chew on grass or twigs, but that is probably more for a purge or for additional roughage. I do grow grass for my cats and they usually do not eat it. They sleep in it! If they do eat grass, it is usually thrown back up.

> *Sam: **What I wouldn't give for some nice big taters.***
> *Gollum: **What's taters, precious?***
> *Sam: **Po-ta-toes. Boil 'em, mash 'em, put 'em in a stew.***
> *Nice big golden chips with a piece of fried fish.***
> *Gollum spits*
> *Sam: **Even you couldn't say no to that.***
> *Gollum: **Oh yes we could! Spoilin' nice fish.***
> *Give it to us raw and wigglin'. You keep nasty chips!***
> *Sam: **You're hopeless.***

-- The Lord of the Rings - The Two Towers

While adding vegetables to a cat's diet may not cause urinary tract or dental problems, it is probably better to choose a fiber source that does not add carbohydrates to the diet or is not alkaline in nature. This is why I use psyllium husk powder as a form of fiber. It is one of the few sources of fiber that adds no carbohydrates, artificial flavoring, or additives. My cats eat their food better now that it contains no vegetables and I have noticed less refusal factor in cats switching to a raw diet that does not contain vegetables.

Fiber

Fiber is also referred to as roughage or bulk — the body cannot digest it. Dietary fiber is found in grains, fruits and vegetables. There is virtually no fiber in meat, fish, eggs, or dairy products. The natural foods of cats typically contain less than one percent dietary fiber. Pet food manufacturers will tell you cats *tolerate* higher levels of fiber in their food, but I think I would like to feed my cats something beyond what they *tolerate*. Extra fiber is added to different prescription diets and other formulas like hairball control in an effort to undo the damage that was done to the cat by feeding commercial food.

There are two different kinds of fiber. Soluble fiber can be dissolved in water and inside the small intestine to form a jelly-like bulk. Soluble fiber can be found in foods such as oat bran, apples, citrus, pears, peas, beans and psyllium. Soluble fibers act mostly in the small intestine since they are destroyed in the large intestine through bacterial action.

Insoluble fibers cannot be dissolved in water and are not destroyed by bacteria in the colon. They are found in wheat bran, cabbage and root vegetables. Insoluble fibers work mainly in the colon where they add bulk and help retain water, resulting in a softer and large stool.

Soluble fibers are rapidly broken down (fermented) by bacteria in the large intestine and do not promote bowel movements. Fibers that are insoluble promote laxation and are either slowly or not fermented. Two notable exceptions to these general guidelines are oats, which contain up to 50 percent soluble fiber and psyllium seed husks that also analyze as soluble fiber. Both of these fiber sources promote laxation and modulate gastric and small intestine physiology.

Commercial pet food labels carry an analysis of crude fiber content, usually around 2.5 percent. The analysis of crude fiber substantially underestimates total dietary fiber in all these materials and is not a reliable method for comparing the fiber content of different foodstuffs.

Research on fiber, short chain fatty acids (SCFA), fructooligosaccharides (FOS) and fermentation pertains more to humans and herbivores (who naturally eat food containing high levels of carbohydrates and fiber,) and who have the anatomic ability to digest higher levels of carbohydrates and fiber. Carnivores digest food quite differently than herbivores. Fermentation of fiber by colonic bacteria may yield short chain fatty acids that are an important energy source for cattle and horses but they provide less than 5 percent of the energy needs of dogs and cats because of the short intestinal tract and relatively fast transit time in those species.[87]

Feeding a diet devoid of some form of fiber may result in constipation or an uncomfortably hard stool.

I have used psyllium husk powder as fiber in my cats' diet for many years now. You may hear some cautions about long-term use of psyllium or use of psyllium in diabetic cats. My cats have suffered no ill health from the use of psyllium and in her paper on diabetic cats which I discussed in Chapter 2, Dr. Greco recommends using psyllium to increase fiber in the diet instead of using a prescription high fiber diet because many cats find prescription high fiber diets unpalatable.

Chapter 12 - Parasites and Other Nasties

The more common feline worms – round worms and tape worms are a fact of life and generally do not mean their host harm. The worms are dependent upon the host for their room and board. An unhealthy cat will suffer from infestation with worms. Worms can cause problems in young kittens. Cats eating commercial food get worms — raw food does not cause worms. A cat hunting and consuming prey may contract worms.

Unlike most people who feed a raw meat diet, I will not say I have never had worms or other parasites in my cats. I have had roundworm infestations in a few cats. It never caused me any concern until Yukon threw up a belly full of live worms all over my couch. It was incredibly nasty and I freaked out when I saw him do it. After I calmed down, I de-wormed him and never had to do it again. It was a sign of Yukon's good health that he expelled all of these live worms instead of dead worms passing through his digestive system in dribs and drabs.

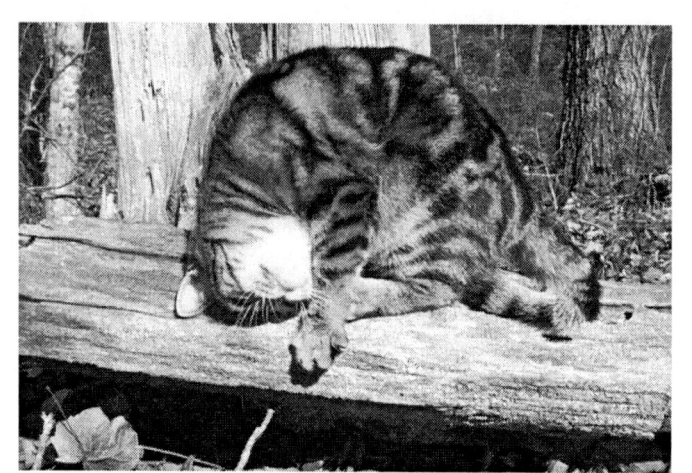

If a cat has worms, then he should be de-wormed. Do not de-worm your cat on a routine basis. Have a fecal test done twice a year if you are concerned about worms. I have never used holistic de-worming medicine. Although I recognize conventional de-worming medicine is toxic, I have never had to worm a cat more than once. Use a brand your holistic veterinarian recommends.

Salmonella and Eschericia coli

Cats are not prone to salmonella or E.coli because of their anatomy. They have short, acidic digestive systems. Food passes through a cat's system quicker than a human's. Table 10 details intestine length and retention time. The retention time for a cat is very short – humans retain food twice as long as a cat! Food does not sit around in a cat's digestive system allowing bacteria to reproduce.

Table 10 – Intestinal Lengths of a Dog, Cat and Human

	Dog	Cat	Human
Small Intestine (meters)	3.9	1.7	7.0
Large Intestine (meters)	0.6	0.4	1.8
Total length (meters)	4.5	2.1	8.8
Body length (meters)	0.75	0.5	1.75
Total length:body length (meters)	4-5	3	5
Mean retention time (hours)	22.6 ± 2.2	13	45.6 ± 11.1

Table courtesy of http://www.speedyvet.com

Humans can become ill with salmonella or E.coli because they have longer, more alkaline systems. In general, bacteria survive better in an alkaline pH than an acid pH.

In the almost ten years I have been feeding raw meat to my cats, none have become ill in any manner from the meat. Use some caution in the meat you feed your cats – organic or free range meat is cleaner due to the environment of the animals prior to slaughter. Clean your work surfaces well after making food. A gallon of water, a splash of bleach, white wine vinegar and a biodegradable cleaner will clean and disinfect your surfaces and be safe for your cat and for the environment.

It is prudent to avoid all conventional cleaners around cats – pine cleaners like Lysol are toxic to cats.

In an article written by Patrick L. McDonough, M.S., Ph.D. he states that,

"Clinical salmonellosis in cats is relatively uncommon and few references to it exist in the scientific literature.

Cats appear to be highly resistant to salmonella infection unless they are stressed by overcrowding, dietary changes, transport, hospitalization, antimicrobial therapy, or concurrent illness at the time of salmonella exposure. The source of the salmonella is most likely to be either contaminated feed, water, or carrier animals (whether clinically ill or healthy). Contamination can arise from rodent or bird feces, raw or undercooked or contaminated meat and table scraps, or commercially prepared foods that are contaminated during processing."[88]

Toxoplasmosis

Toxoplasma gondii is an intracellular parasite and is one of the most common parasitic diseases of animals and man. The definitive hosts for the parasite (the only animals in which organism reproduces sexually) are members of the *Felidae* family. Infection with *T gondii* is extremely common, but rarely a cause of significant disease in any species.[89]

Cats exposed to *T gondii* usually begin shedding cysts between 3 and 10 days after ingestion of infected tissue and continue shedding for around 10-14 days, during which time many millions of cysts may be produced. Once a cat has developed an immune response, further shedding of cysts is extremely rare.[90]

Although there is a high prevalence of infection in cats, most surveys show a less than 1% incidence of cyst shedding. This is to be expected as infected cats generally do not re-shed cysts following their first exposure to *T gondii*.[91]

Significant clinical disease in cats (and other species) appears to be very rare. When disease does occur, it may develop either following primary infection or as a result of reactivated infection (where compromised immunity allows the reactivation of infection).[92]

Pregnant women and individuals with an autoimmune disease like AIDS or cancer should use caution when handling raw meat and cleaning the litter box. A cat that has a compromised immune system may not develop immunity to *T gondii* and may continue shedding the parasitic cysts. Work with a competent homeopathic veterinarian to improve the health if you believe his immune system to be compromised.

Diligent litter box cleaning is important to avoid infection. Remove stool from your cat's litter box at least daily (if not several times during the day). Use disposable rubber gloves if you are pregnant or suffering from an immunosuppressive disease. Keep children away from your cat's litter box.

If you plan to become pregnant in the near future, have a blood test done to see if you have been previously exposed to toxoplasmosis and have developed toxoplasmosis antibodies. If you have, you can relax. If you do not have antibodies, then use caution when handling raw meat and cleaning the litter box. A study in the *New England Journal of Medicine* showed no correlation between cat ownership and infection with toxoplasmosis.[93][94]

I have never used food grade hydrogen peroxide or grape seed extract to presoak the meat I feed my cats. I have never been concerned about any type of food poisoning in my cats or myself. I do not want to soak my cats' meat because I do not want to lose any blood from the meat.

If you feed human grade raw meat from a quality source, your cats *should* be fine. I emphasize *should* because if your cats are stressed by overcrowding, dietary changes, transport, or hospitalization they may be at risk, no matter what they are fed. Cats treated with excessive antibiotics or steroids are at risk as are those with immunosuppressive diseases.

> *"Security is mostly superstition. It does not exist in nature ... Avoiding danger is no safer in the long run than outright exposure. The fearful are caught as often as the bold."*
> -- Helen Adams Keller

Chapter 13 - Diet Polish – Supplements to Round Out the Balance

The meat that we purchase in a grocery store or at butcher is usually not raised in a natural manner. Even meat that is labeled organic is usually from animals that are fed grain. Unless the meat is labeled "grass-fed" or something you raise yourself, the following supplements are necessary. A cat's natural prey would be animals eating their natural food namely grasses and seeds. Animals consuming grass and seeds are naturally higher in protein, lower in fat, higher in omega 3 fatty acids and other vitamins such as vitamin E. It is necessary to add the following supplements to the meat you feed your cat in order to bring the nutritional value of the meat closer to wild meat. In a perfect world all animals would be raised in a natural manner. They would be healthy and those animals raised for food would be healthier for those consuming them.

This recipe is very similar in ingredients and proportions to the one presented in Feline Future's *The Backyard Predator*.[95]

Water

It is imperative that you add at least a cup of spring or filtered water to the diet if you are using psyllium husk powder. Yerba Prima, a manufacturer of psyllium husk powder, recommends eight ounces of water for every teaspoon of psyllium husk powder. Since the recipe contains two teaspoons of psyllium husk, according to Yerba Prima, sixteen ounces of water should be added, however, that makes for a very soupy mixture. You can add more water to the food prior to serving if desired.

The more ground meat that is in the recipe, the more water you can get into the mixture without it becoming soup. Alternatively, the more chunks of meat in the mixture, the thicker you want the supplement mixture to be so it sticks to the food.

A creature will perish from lack of water long before it will die from starvation. Cats evolved as desert creatures. They obtain much of their necessary water intake from their prey that is between 65-75 percent water.

There is a misconception that cats on a raw diet do not drink water. A cat does not have to drink water while eating a raw diet because there is sufficient water in the food, but they do still drink water if it is available to them. Kittens do tend to drink more than adults.

Excessive water consumption, especially when on a raw diet, is cause for concern. If your cat is constantly hanging out by the water bowl and is urinating frequently, you should probably have a blood test done to test kidney function. This becomes more of a concern as a cat ages.

You may notice your cat may urinate *more* (not more frequently, the volume of urine may increase). I believe this is due to the cat receiving more water in his food with this type of diet. Dry food is less than 10 percent water. Even if a cat drinks water on his own, a cat consuming dry food is still not getting the hydration he needs to remain healthy.

> *"The highest goodness is like water. Water benefits all things and does not compete. It stays in the lowly places which others despise. Therefore it is near The Eternal."*
> *-- Lao Tzo*

Water is very important to all living creatures. I believe sufficient water intake is more important to skin and coat condition than oils. My cats all have beautiful coats and the only oil that is in their diet is salmon oil. I normally do not bathe my cats prior to showing them. They do not need to be bathed — their coats are shiny and silky day in and day out. That is the first thing people notice about my cats is their coat. If oil or fat was so important to coat condition I do not think my cats on such a low fat diet would have such nice coats. If someone asks me about adding additional oils to their cat's diet to improve coat, I advise them to increase the water in the diet.

Do not give your cat tap water. It may contain minerals or toxins your cat may be sensitive to. Use spring or filtered water. If you use well water, have it tested periodically for high mineral content or use a filter.

For one recipe use at least one cup of spring or filtered water.

Egg Yolk

Whole eggs represent the most complete and concentrated nutrition available in the animal kingdom. The egg white contains most of the protein and amino acids with the egg yolk containing most of the vitamins and fatty acids.

There is a protein in egg whites called avidin that binds with biotin and inhibits absorption in many animals including cats. Avidin is known as an anti-vitamin. In order for this to occur, an excessive number of raw eggs must be consumed over a period of time. The major sign of biotin deficiency in virtually all species is scaly, dry dermatitis. Long antibiotic (especially sulfa antibiotics) use can also induce a biotin deficiency.

Carey and Morris produced biotin deficiency by including 18.5 to 32 percent egg white in a purified diet fed to eight-week-old kittens. It took 150 days to see signs of deficiency.[96] I recognize that is a lot of egg white over an extended period of time, but I have been unable to find information that makes me feel comfortable feeding egg whites on a daily basis, therefore, I recommend feeding just the yolks. Even if there is sufficient biotic in the yolk, if a protein in the white *interferes* with absorption of biotin, it would not matter how much biotin was in the egg yolk or the rest of the diet for that matter.

Of course a wild cat raiding a nest of eggs would eat the whole egg, however, eggs are not the staple of a wild cat's diet. If whole eggs were used in the recipe detailed in this book and fed on a daily basis, the egg whites may indeed cause a problem with biotin absorption. Feeding whole eggs as a meal on an occasional basis should not be a problem for your cat.

Use good quality eggs. If you can get eggs from hens that are free range or fed a vegetarian diet, those are the best to use.

Use two raw egg yolks per recipe.

Psyllium Husk Powder

Two teaspoons of psyllium husk powder are added as a form of fiber. Fiber assists in moving your cat's food through his digestive system. A diet without fiber would result in stools that are dry and difficult to pass. A cat's natural form of fiber would be his prey's hide or feathers. Raw bone also provides some fiber.

You must add at least a cup of water to the recipe otherwise it will lead to constipation. Use the powdered form of psyllium husk which is a more concentrated form of fiber, not the whole husk or seeds.

Be careful when you are mixing up the powder. Some people are sensitive to the dust from psyllium husk powder.

Use two teaspoons of psyllium husk powder per recipe.

Salmon Oil

Salmon oil is added as a source of omega 3 fatty acids, namely eicosapentaenoic acid (EPA) and docosahexaenoic acid (DHA). EPA is naturally occurring in the tissues of animals consuming grass and seeds. DHA is naturally occurring in the brains and eyes of the prey animal. Of all the fish oils, salmon oil is the most concentrated form of EPA and DHA. Do not use cod liver as a fatty acid supplement as it is high in vitamins A and D. I use Carlson brand which has a very high level of EPA and DHA per capsule. Two capsules of Carlson provide 360 mg of EPA and 250 mg DHA.

I do not recommend using salmon oil in any form other than that in individual capsules. Salmon oil is particularly sensitive to oxidation. Any exposure to air will cause the oil to turn rancid.

Use 2,000 mg salmon oil (usually two capsules) per recipe.

Kelp and Dulse

As you will see in Table 9, kelp and dulse are added as a source of minerals such as iron, niacin and potassium that are deficient in conventionally raised meat. Blue green algae is not a substitute for sea vegetables. Because kelp is particularly high in iodine, do not use more than a teaspoon of kelp in a recipe.

You should purchase kelp and dulse in powdered or granulated form. Mix them together in a large container and store it in a cool, dry place.

Use 1 teaspoon of a mixture of kelp and dulse if you are using the meat with bone recipe, 2 teaspoons of the mixture of you are not using bone. *Do not* use all kelp – it contains too much iodine. If you cannot find dulse, use just one teaspoon of kelp in the recipe.

Table 9 - Nutritional Analysis of Various Sea Vegetables

	ALARIA	DULSE	KELP	NORI	
PROTEIN g/100gms	17.7	21.5	16.1	28.4	57g*
FAT g/100gms	3.6	1.7	2.4	4.5	77g*
CARBOHYDRATE g/100gms	39.8	44.6	39.3	45.1	345g*
CALORIES cal/100g	262	264	241	318	2300 cal*
CALCIUM mg/100g C	1100	213	942	168	800mgs†
POTASSIUM mg/100g K	7460	7820	11200	2690	1875-5625mgs††
MAGNESIUM mg/100g Mg	918	271	900	378	350mgs†
PHOSPHOROUS mg/100g P	503	408	423	408	800mgs†
IRON mg/100g Fe	18.1	33.1	42.6	20.9	10mgs†
SODIUM mg/100g Na	4240	1740	4460	1610	1100-3300mgs††
IODINE mg/100g I	16.6	5.2	144	1.4	.15mgs†
MANGANESE mg/100g Mn	1.02	1.14	1.23	3.46	2.5-5mgs††
COPPER mg/100g Cu	0.172	0.376	0.148	0.612	2-3mgs††
CHROMIUM mg/100g Cr	0.21	0.15	0.24	0.12	.05-.20mgs††
FLUORIDE mg/100g F	4.3	5.3	3.9	5.8	1.5-4mgs††
ZINC mg/100g Zn	3.44	2.86	2.86	4.15	15mgs†
VIT A I.U. V-A	8487	663	561	4288	5000 I.U.†
VIT B1 I.U. V-B1	0.558	0.073	0.549	0.577	1.4mgs†
VIT B2 I.U. V-B2	2.73	1.91	2.48	2.93	1.6mgs†
VIT B3 I.U. V-B3	10.5	1.89	3.62	5.92	18mgs†
VIT B6 I.U. V-B6	6.23	8.99	8.63	11.21	2.2mgs†
VIT B12 I.U. V-B12	5.03	6.6	2.6	17.5	3mcgs†
VIT C I.U. V-C	5.9	6.34	4.16	12.08	60mgs†
VIT E I.U. V-E	4.92	1.71	2.71	5.09	15 I.U.†

Table courtesy of Maine Coast Sea Vegetables, **http://www.seaveg.com**

Bone Meal

You need to add bone meal or another form of calcium to the diet *if you do not use raw ground bone*. It is far superior to use ground bone instead of bone meal or other calcium substitute. Use bone meal made for human consumption or a high quality product for pets like Solid Gold. For a recipe you will need to use two tablespoons of bone meal. The bone meal you use should be approximately 22 to 26 percent calcium and 11 percent phosphorus. Bone meal is the best substitute for bone because the calcium is bound with phosphorus like real bone and contains trace minerals.

There are many different calcium substitutes available like calcium carbonate, calcium citrate and calcium lactate. To provide a calculation for every different kind of substitute would be exhausting because they are all different as are the various brands. If you cannot use bone meal and want to use a different calcium substitute, use the excellent calcium/phosphorus converter on-line at **http://www.dataweb.net/~sham/nutrient/index.html**

Gelatin

Gelatin needs to be added *if you do not use raw ground bone* to make up for nutrients lacking in calcium supplements like bone meal. Gelatin is made from calf and cattle skins, de-mineralized cattle bones (ossein) and pork skin and is a rich a source of amino acids that would naturally occur in raw bone.

Use one tablespoon of unflavored gelatin per recipe.

Glandulars

It is thought that ingestion of glandular material of a certain animal gland will strengthen the corresponding gland of the consumer. In the case of infection and immune system deficiencies, thymus extracts and spleen extracts have been found to be quite useful in humans. Use a good quality multi-glandular formula that contains as many different glands as possible. Look for a source that uses organs from bovine sources that are grass-fed on rangeland free of pesticides and fertilizers and from animals where no growth hormones, additives or antibiotics are used.

Some people have been unable to source glandulars, especially those individuals who are in countries other than the United States. If so, they can be omitted from the recipe. If you can source individual glandulars, look for kidney and adrenal as I believe those are the most beneficial for cats. Lifesvigor.com still carries multi-glandulars at a reasonable price.

Use 2 capsules glandulars (or one daily human dose) per recipe.

Vitamin E

Vitamin E helps preserve the meat and prevents its oxidation when exposed to the air during grinding and storage. I use dry vitamin E capsules because they are easier to open than the gel caps.

Freezing or storage for any length of time will destroy the vitamin E in the food. Vitamin E is also destroyed by heat. If you grind and freeze your cat's food for longer than a week or two, you should add an additional pinch of vitamin E to your cat's food once it has defrosted.

Use 400 IU vitamin E per recipe.

Vitamin B

Cats have a particular need for vitamin B3 (niacin) because they do not convert niacin from tryptophan. A cat's niacin requirement is four times that of dogs.[97] In addition, a cat's requirement for vitamin B6 (pyridoxine) is also four times that of dogs.[98] The B vitamins, biotin, vitamin B2 (riboflavin), niacin and pyridoxine are important for healthy skin. Meat and egg yolks are high in B vitamins, however, the addition of 50 mg of vitamin B complex helps your cat maintain a healthy nervous system and combat daily stress. B vitamins are water-soluble and should be replenished daily.

If you feel your cat is going to be exposed to a particularly high level of stress, then double the amount of vitamin B complex in the recipe.

Vitamin B complex consists of several vitamins that are grouped together because of the loose similarities in their properties, distribution in natural sources, and physiological functions. You should use a vitamin B complex that contains a combination of the following B vitamins in a 50 mg. capsule: vitamin B-1 (thiamin), vitamin B-2 (riboflavin), vitamin B-3 (niacin), vitamin B-6, vitamin B-5 (pantothenic acid), vitamin B-12, biotin, folic acid, choline and inositol.

Use 50 mg. vitamin B complex per recipe.

Chapter 14 - Recipe With Bone

This recipe is very similar in ingredients and proportions to the one presented in Feline Future's *The Backyard Predator*.[99]

Approximately two and one-half pounds of meat with bone.

One-half pound (200 grams) raw heart from the same species of animal the muscle meat comes from. If you absolutely cannot source heart substitute 2,000 mg taurine. Note: if you do not use heart, add an additional one-half pound (200 grams) of meat. If you are concerned about loss of taurine due to freezing, feel free to add 2,000 mg of taurine even if you are using raw heart. It is probably over-kill, but it will not harm your cat.

One-quarter pound (or 100 grams) raw liver from the same species of animal the muscle meat comes from. If you absolutely cannot source liver substitute vitamin A/D capsules. You will want approximately 20,000 IU vitamin A and whatever amount of vitamin D comes in the capsule for each recipe. Vitamin A/D capsules usually come in amounts of 10,000 IU vitamin A and 400 IU vitamin D per capsule. You can also use 2 tablespoons of cod liver oil, however, cod liver oil goes rancid quite quickly. I prefer the dry vitamin A/D capsules. Note: if you do not use liver, add an additional one-quarter pound (100 grams) of meat.

> If you are feeding rabbit or turkey and cannot source rabbit or turkey liver or heart, substitute chicken liver or heart. These substitutions are not ideal, but it is better than using supplemental taurine and vitamins A and D.

2 high-quality raw egg yolks

2 teaspoons psyllium husk powder; if you are using whole psyllium husk pods, use 4 teaspoons

1 cup (or more) spring (or filtered) water

2,000 mg salmon oil (usually 2 capsules)

1 teaspoon kelp and dulse combined; *do not* use all kelp. If you cannot source dulse, use just one-half to one teaspoon of kelp

50 mg. vitamin B complex

400 IU vitamin E

2 glandular capsules

Preparation: remove as much skin from chicken or turkey as you can. Cut as much meat off the bone as you can and cut it into chunks the size that your cat will eat. Mine are approximately quarter-sized. Put the chunks in the bowl.

Grind the heart and liver into the same bowl the chunks of meat are. Then grind the bone. Run the salmon oil capsules through the grinder with the meat. This eliminates the need to prick the capsule to express the oil out. It is safe for your cat to consume the capsules.

Gently mix to combine.

In a separate bowl add the egg yolks, water, psyllium husk powder, salmon oil (if not run through grinder), vitamin B complex, vitamin E and glandulars. The taurine and vitamin A/D capsules (if used) should be added as well. Mix well with a whisk. Gently fold the supplement mixture into meat. Divide the mixture into serving packages and freeze or refrigerate.

Chapter 15 - Recipe Without Bone

This recipe is very similar in ingredients and proportions to the one presented in Feline Future's *The Backyard Predator*.[100]

Approximately one and a half pounds of muscle meat.

One-half pound (200 grams) raw heart from the same species of animal the muscle meat comes from. If you absolutely cannot source heart substitute 2,000 mg taurine. Note: if you do not use heart, add an additional one-half pound (200 grams) of meat. If you are concerned about loss of taurine due to freezing, feel free to add 2,000 mg of taurine even if you are using raw heart. It is probably over-kill, but it will not harm your cat.

One-quarter pound (100 grams) raw liver from the same species of animal the muscle meat comes from. If you absolutely cannot source liver substitute vitamin A/D capsules. You will want approximately 20,000 IU vitamin A and whatever amount of vitamin D comes in the capsule for each recipe. Vitamin A/D capsules usually come in amounts of 10,000 IU vitamin A and 400 IU vitamin D per capsule. You can also use 2 tablespoons of cod liver oil, however, cod liver oil goes rancid quite quickly. I prefer the dry vitamin A/D capsules. Note: if you do not use liver, add an additional one-quarter pound (100 grams) of meat.

> If you are using rabbit or turkey and cannot source rabbit or turkey liver or heart, use chicken liver or heart. These substitutions are not ideal, but it is better than using supplemental taurine and vitamins A and D.

> If you are using lamb and cannot source lamb heart or liver, use beef or calf heart or liver. These substitutions are not ideal, but it is better than using supplemental taurine and vitamins A and D.

2 tablespoons bone meal (human grade or high quality pet grade, not the bone meal you can buy in a garden supply store)

1 tablespoon unflavored gelatin

2 high-quality raw egg yolks

2 teaspoons psyllium husk powder; if you are using psyllium husk pods, use 4 teaspoons

1 cup (or more) spring (or filtered) water

2,000 mg salmon oil (usually 2 capsules)

2 teaspoons kelp and dulse combined; *do not* use all kelp. If you cannot source dulse, use just 1 teaspoon of kelp

50 mg. vitamin B complex

400 IU vitamin E

2 glandular capsules

Preparation: cut at least half the muscle meat into chunks and put them in the bowl.

Grind what muscle meat you did not chunk, heart and liver into the same bowl the chunks of meat are. Run the salmon oil capsules through the grinder with the meat. This eliminates the need to prick the capsule to express the oil out. It is safe for your cat to consume the capsules.

Gently mix to combine.

In a separate bowl add the bone meal, gelatin, egg yolks, water, psyllium husk powder, salmon oil (if not run through grinder), vitamin B complex, vitamin E and glandulars. The taurine and vitamin A/D capsules (if used) should be added as well. Mix well with a whisk. Gently fold into meat. Divide the mixture into serving packages and freeze or refrigerate.

Chapter 16 - Time Saving Tips

- Partially freeze the meat prior to processing it. You will find the skin comes off easily and you can cut the meat off the bone and chunk it more easily. It also clogs less in the grinder if it is partially frozen.

- Buy your liver and heart in bulk (if you can) and package them in zipper-type sandwich bags in portions of 100 grams of liver, 200 grams of heart. Freeze and defrost as needed. Do not discard the blood from the organ meat — use it in your recipe.

- Make up several recipes of dry supplements and store them in an airtight container. I will often make as many as 30-50 recipes at one time. In case you want to do this, here's the break down for ten recipes of supplement to use with the meat with bone recipe:

    6 tablespoons + 2 teaspoons psyllium husk powder

    6 tablespoons + 2 teaspoons seaweed mixture (note half and half kelp and dulse or a mixture of kelp and dulse)

    10 capsules 50 mg. vitamin B complex or 5 capsules 100 mg. vitamin B complex

    10 capsules 400 IU dry vitamin E

    20 capsules glandulars

    Open all the capsules and put in a large container with a cover. Shake well.

    For one recipe use approximately 2 tablespoons powder.

- Use poultry shears instead of a knife to cut meat off the bone and chunking.

- Cover your work surface and surrounding walls if necessary with newspaper to ease clean-up.

- Run the salmon oil capsules through the grinder when you grind the meat. That eliminates the need to poke them to get the oil out. Run some meat through the grinder <u>before</u> the salmon oil capsules, otherwise it will squirt out all over the place and make a smelly mess.

- Put serving portions of your finished mixture on a flexible cutting board. Use the flexible cutting board to pour the mixture into a zip lock bag or other container for storage.

- Run a few ice cubes or a slice of toasted bread through the grinder when you are through grinding to clean out any remaining meat. I prefer ice cubes because I let them fall right into the bowl of meat. I do not want toasted bread in my cat food.

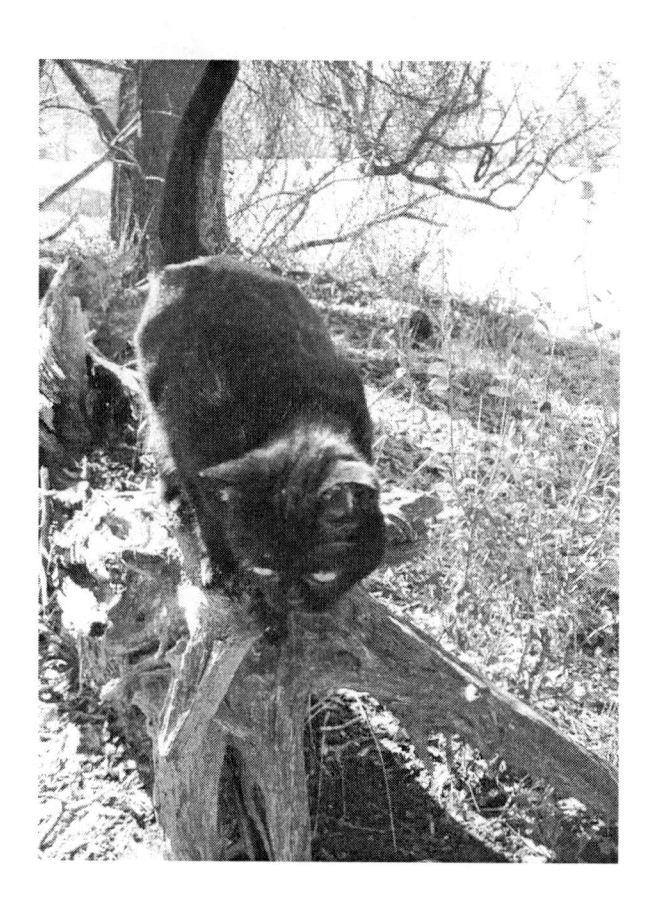

Chapter 17 - Serving Tips

There is a lot of confusion on how much to feed a cat per meal. I do not know how much my cats eat in a meal. They are all different. They also eat more on some days than on others. For example, they usually eat less in the warmer months than they do in the cold months. One half-cup per meal per cat is a good place to start. If your cat eats a full half-cup and is looking for more, let him have it. Let him eat as much as he wants for 30 minutes, then put any leftovers in the refrigerator.

I feed my cats at least twice a day. Whenever possible, I feed them three times a day. Since a small cat can only kill small prey, they need to eat quite frequently in the wild. Do not leave the food down for longer than 30 minutes.

Kittens, pregnant and nursing females and very old cats will need to eat more frequently. I feed my kittens four to five times a day until they are four months old, four times a day until they are six months old and then two or three times a day from then on. Pregnant cats in their third trimester and nursing cats are fed at least four times a day.

Cats will often be extremely enthusiastic about their food when it is first prepared only to turn their noses up at it when the same food is offered the next day. This is not unusual. If your healthy cat does not want to eat a meal or two or even three, do not worry. If your cat is acting normal in all respects except for not wanting to eat for a day or two, that is fine. A day or two without food will not harm a healthy cat. They can be fussbudgets about eating. I have a few who do not care for chicken, they like rabbit, but often will not eat chicken a day or two after it has been prepared. Use caution in fasting an unhealthy or overweight cat. If your cat has been consuming commercial food, he is at greater risk of developing fatty liver disease.

If your cat is not feeling well and does not want to eat a meal or two, respect that decision on the part of your cat. A fast allows your cat to pool healing resources – digestion uses considerable resources.

You should put effort into making food for your cat, but if he does not eat the same amount every meal or refuses a meal, do not worry *as long as he is acting normal*.

If your cat is refusing food for longer than a couple of days and not acting right, then you may want to contact a veterinarian, preferably one that is holistic.

Gently warm your cat's food prior to serving. *Do not* microwave it. I put mine in a cheap gallon-size plastic bag then soak it in a hot water bath for about 15 minutes. This warms the food without cooking it. Partially cooking the food could cause your cat to throw it back up.

Cats vomit easily — that is part of their nature, they have short digestive systems. Do not be too concerned if your cat occasionally vomits his food. Sometimes they eat too fast. If you have a cat that is gorging on his food, make the chunks larger. If that does not work, offer very small portions at a time. Sometimes they will try to swallow a chunk of meat that is too large. Yukon does this all the time. I have yet to have a cat choke to death on a piece of meat.

Sometimes I have to rescue a couple of my cats that temporarily forget they have teeth that are supposed to cut the food into manageable pieces. The dingy cat would sit there with a hunk of meat hanging out of her mouth chewing away for hours. Sometimes they'll even start running around the house in a frenzy – maybe they think speed will assist in chewing the meat? Some of my more intelligent cats have figured out that they can hold one end of the piece of meat with a claw and pull on it with their teeth in order to "cut" it. Usually my female cats are smarter than my males, but when it comes to figuring out how to consume a large piece of meat, the prize goes to my males. Perhaps the females do not want to use their claws to hold meat because they do not want get their paws dirty.

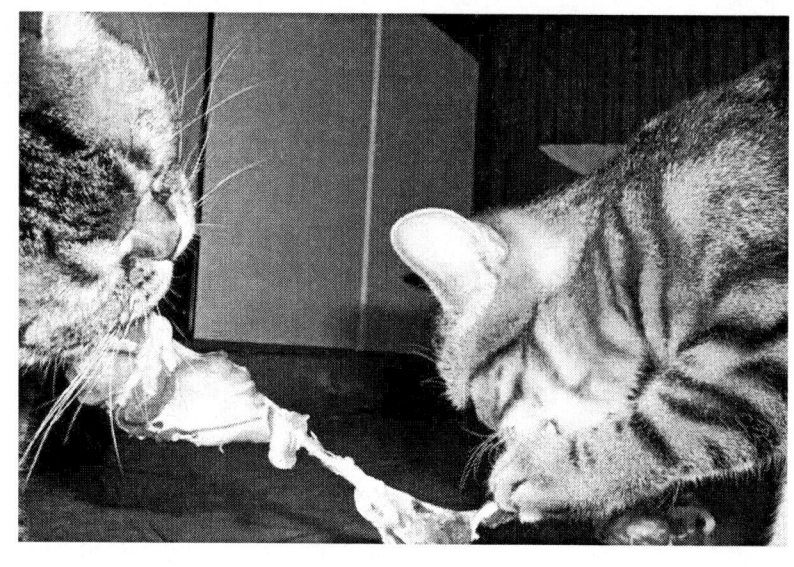

Do not be concerned. Your cats will figure out how to consume their food.

I believe cats prefer eating off a plate instead of a bowl. I usually use paper plates to feed my cats. My cats do make a mess in the kitchen when they eat. Wiley would often bring a piece of meat into the TV room to eat with me. It was his form of a TV dinner. If you have a cat that insists on dragging food around the house, you may need to confine him during feeding time. If you have carpet in your kitchen, you can purchase a piece of heavy-grade plastic to put down on the carpet to protect it.

Chapter 18 - Switching Reluctant Cats

I have not had difficulty switching a cat to a raw food diet since I first started out with Pumpkin. If I had known what I know today, things would have gone differently. If you have a cat that absolutely will not eat raw food, then I suggest having a homeopathic work-up done. Dr. Levy gave me a good piece of advice back when I was so upset about Pumpkin's refusal to eat, "a healthy cat will eat anything." He is right. Addiction or intolerance to any type of species-appropriate food is a sign of ill health and it should be addressed.

Cats can be quite stubborn when it comes to trying a new food. They get very attached to the type and texture of food they were weaned on. Pet food manufacturers have done a brilliant job in making their food palatable to cats. Open a bag of dry food and take a whiff. You will know why cats are attracted to it. It is highly scented and flavored. I often think commercial cat food contains some secret ingredient to addict cats.

Some cats switch to a raw food diet without going on a hunger strike. Usually young cats are easier to convert than older cats. Kittens naturally gravitate to raw food – they know what is good for them! If you have a young cat that is *healthy*, I think switching the "cold turkey" method is acceptable, however, it is advisable to enlist the help of a holistic veterinarian during the process, just in case. A 24 to 48 hour fast is not in any way harmful for a young *healthy* cat. Do not fast an old, overweight, or ill cat without the support of a holistic veterinarian. I reiterate what I have said numerous times throughout this book — try to find a holistic veterinarian to support you if you are planning on switching your cat to a more natural lifestyle. Most conventional veterinarians are not going to support this decision. If you cat has been consuming commercial food, he is at greater risk of developing fatty liver disease.

If you expect you are going to have a battle on your hands I suggest not making a full recipe of food. Offer small pieces of raw chicken, turkey, lamb, or beef to your cat to see what he may prefer. I have found many cats prefer poultry to beef or lamb. Once you know what type of meat he prefers, then make up a recipe and divide it into very small serving portions and freeze them. There is no sense wasting meat and supplements on a cat that is going to be initially fussy.

I suggest if your cat has been eating dry food and you are feeding your cat on a free choice basis that you first take up the food and feed the cat on a schedule. Feed him twice a day and only leave the food down about 30 minutes. After the 30 minutes is up, put away the food. You should store the dry food in a completely air tight container preferably somewhere out of the house. Cats have a highly developed sense of smell. If they can smell the dry food in the house, they will hold out for it.

Once your cat is eating on a schedule you will notice that he is excited about food. That is a good sign. You can try to offer raw food at this point. You may be pleasantly surprised. I think when cats have food left in front of them 24/7 they tend to lose enthusiasm for their food. If you had a particular type of smelly food left in front of you all the time you would not be too interested in that food either. If your cat only licks the food or eats only a tiny bit, you are home free – he is accepting what you have put in front of him as "food."

> *"Just don't give up trying to do what you really want to do.*
> *Where there is love and inspiration, I don't think you can go wrong."*
> *-- Ella Fitzgerald*

Another option for a cat eating dry food is to try Wysong's Archetype food. Archetype is a cold-processed dried food that is 99 percent meat and contains no grains. The Wysong products make a good transition food.

A cat that is eating canned food may be a bit easier to convert than one eating dry food. Mix a very small amount of raw food into the canned. As with the method above, if you cat refuses to eat during one meal, he should eat for the next meal.

I have not personally known of a suicidal cat. They usually are very much into self-preservation – *most cats* will not starve themselves to death. They will put forth their best effort to convince you that they are being horribly mistreated and are about to die, but do not believe them. Cats can be very stubborn about what they consider to be "food." Dry food junkies can be the worst. You have to be as stubborn as your cat. You have to be sure in your mind you are doing the right thing – believe me, you are. For the most part, cats do not remain healthy on commercial food for any length of time. Eventually the problems associated with feeding commercial cat food are going to catch up with your cat. It is not optimal food – it is like you eating a steady diet of potato chips instead of fresh potatoes that you cook yourself.

A sick cat or one in a stressed environment like a shelter or hospital may be in danger of starving to death. That is different than your household companion. I cannot tell you in good conscience to switch a reluctant cat "cold turkey." If it were my cat it would be different and I probably would switch him cold turkey. I do not know your cat and I am not there to observe him. Most cats do switch to a raw food diet within 48 hours if offered nothing else to eat. You have to do what is right for you and your cat. Be patient and persistent and you will get there.

There are a number of bribe foods you can try to mix into the raw food such as Wysong's F-Biotic supplement, or their canned all-meat product, canned tuna (or other fish) juice, meat baby food, Tuna Dash, heavy cream, grated cheese, or juicy cooked meat.

I have seen a lot less refusal factor with this type of diet. I believe it is because there are no ingredients in the diet that cats really do not care for like vegetables, grains and vitamin C. I know my cats eat this type of diet better than they did when I fed grains and vegetables.

Here is some advice from the pros:

"It took 7-8 months to switch Emilie. For months, she did not even admit it was food - treated it like a pile of dirt. Wouldn't so much as lick it. I kept putting it in front of her, she'd turn up her nose. I would put it away and feed her something else. Over and over! Possibly I should have met her refusal with more resolve! Finally, one day, I decided to drizzle a bit of tuna juice over it. Bingo! Cleaned up a whole plate. I was in awe! Then, I began to top it off with a bit of Wellness or Wysong canned ... the glorious moment came when I caught her eating AROUND the canned! Usually, she'll dig right in - occasionally, I still have to top it a bit. We now have 2 raw eating machines here - feels good!"

- Joanna from the Natural Cat List

****

"I tried once to switch my cats, gave up and then tried again several months later. I did it very gradually using Wellness canned food — mostly Wellness and a little bit of raw, gradually (very gradually) phasing out the canned food until it was all raw. Now they won't eat canned!!"

- Terry from the Natural Cat List

****

"Well I am still switching a reluctant cat, but it is getting easier. At first she looked at me like I was trying to kill her. I tried cooking the food, cooking chicken and adding it, adding tuna, adding catnip and many other things. I was getting fed up and I think that she was beginning to lose weight. I refused to give in and she refused to budge. Please do not think me cruel, but I also tried force-feeding her, I felt guilty but it did get her to try it of her own will for two seconds. As a last resort, I took her to the bathroom and tried feeding her a whole quail leg. I was shocked when she decided to eat it. The only thing that I can get her to happily eat is quail and luckily it is cheap here in Vancouver.

For the raw diet the thing that finally worked was adding a little bit of her old canned cat food. The raw food disappeared. The food itself is in little cubes so I crushed them and mixed them very well with the raw food. Now she is happy to see the bag of raw food come out of the fridge. I slowly phased out the canned food."

- Kelly Sassy and Smudge from the Natural Cat List

****

"It took me a while to even remember that I had experienced problems switching. In fact, I got a good laugh remembering. I only had 3 cats at the time. I put the raw food down on the floor for the second time. It was ignored by all 3 the first time. Bunny Rabbit came over and gave it a sniff, dropped her ears back, crouched down and hissed at me. When I reached out to her she swatted at me and ran upstairs and hid under the dresser. I tried to get her out but she just howled and hissed. I got frantic and e-mailed Michelle asking her for help. I gave her my phone number and then practically sat on the phone waiting for her call. As you can imagine, she told me to ignore the behavior and wait her out. I thought I had done permanent damage to my little kitty and it was just a snot-ball, temper tantrum. It never occurred to me that a little animal could get such a 'tude. Live and learn. The little brat eats most everything I put down now or she tries to cover it up and goes hungry. Someone once told me that they had forgotten more than I would ever learn and I thought to myself, "what an old poop you are!" But now I know what he meant. As life goes on you actually forget what you did not know and how the lack of knowledge made you behave."

— Bev from the Natural Cat list

****

"I still remember it well and compared to many folks, our switch was pretty easy. The first time I served up a huge plate of raw, both cats wolfed it down and then I thought, 'hey, I have got this thing licked.' Then I panicked that maybe all those anti-raw folks were right and I'd killed my cats. I followed them around like a mother hen for the next day waiting for them to keel over. But they did not. But the next day when I served it they both looked at me as if I were deranged. No WAY were they going to eat this stuff. So I just re-started VERY small by adding about 1/3 tsp. of raw food in their coveted canned food and over three weeks, slowly added more until they were all raw. Then I removed the kibble (which actually they'd more or less stopped having an interest in anyway). Duke protested for one day then got over it.

In that vein, I am seriously considering writing myself a 'letter' to save until next spring. It will say something like this: Dear Anne, It's spring again and the cats are probably acting weird. Nettie has gone off her food and you're fretting. Just stop it. This happens EVERY year and if you give it time she will get over it. Do not forget that this ALWAYS happens with the change in weather and stop with all that anxiety already. Love, Anne"

— Anne from the Natural Cat List

****

"I switched my cats cold turkey because they only ate kibble all of their life and they would not eat it on top of the raw. So cold turkey it was. Two of the younger cats had no problem but the two older cats went without food for several days. Finally one of them started on the raw but the last, Shelly, she would not give in. I did put some in her mouth every day. Michelle told me to be careful because that might be the way I would have to feed her forever, by hand. She ate that way for about two weeks I literally had to hold the food in my fingers so she would eat it. After reading what others do to get their cat to eat, tuna juice and canned food, I decided to put the salmon oil directly on top of their food and that has worked ever since. If I forgot to put the salmon oil on top Shelly reminds me by not eating it. Crazy Cat."

— Margaret from the Natural Cat List

Chapter 19 - Success Stories

I have had nothing but success in feeding my cats a raw diet. There have been many people I have met over the years who have switched their cats to a raw diet because they were sick. I hate to think of what some of these cats went through before their caregivers "discovered" raw diet.

It makes me very sad to know these cats did not need to suffer and in some cases die. Here are some of their stories:

"By the time my sweet orange tabby cat Duke (pictured below) was five years old, he had daily diarrhea. A mellow cream puff of a cat, Duke had never had a robust digestive system. As early as his kittenhood, he was gassy and had recurrent bright red spots of red in his watery stools. Our vet did not seem too alarmed and never once questioned my feeding him Science Diet kibble and Nutro-Max canned food. As the years passed, I couldn't help but notice the problem was becoming frequent until one day I realized that my gentle beast was *never* putting out a well-formed stool.

Ultimately, Duke was diagnosed with inflammatory bowel disease (IBD) and the vet sent me home with a pricey bag of prescription kibble. The vet suggested that if this diet "improvement" didn't do the trick, daily prednisone steroid treatments almost always relieved the chronic inflammation that plagued cats with this very common malady. Armed with the new kibble and convinced that would set things right, I watched Duke closely for signs of improvement that never came.

I was instinctively reluctant to sentence him to daily doses of immune-suppressing steroids. Years earlier, I'd lost two very beloved cats to complications from conventional treatment for hyperthyroidism and was still shaken by the experience. I began tentatively researching alternatives. Even though I had an impressive little library of cat books — including books on holistic cat care — I always skipped straight over the chapters that advocated a raw diet for cats because, frankly, the idea seemed absurd, dangerous, and overwhelmingly difficult.

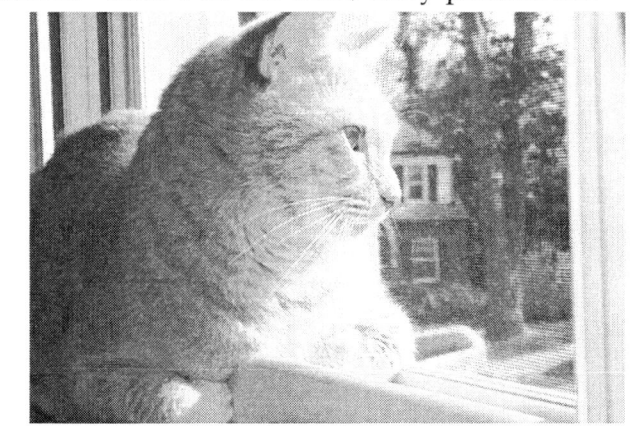

My wake-up call came about two days after Duke went through a routine dental cleaning. It's not clear whether it was the stress of the procedure, the anesthetic, or the unavoidable unleashing of lots of bacteria in his already compromised system, but Duke had an absolutely awful IBD flare-up that required hospitalization. I found him one sad morning crouched in pain and extremely dehydrated from having spent the night vomiting and having at least half a dozen episodes of violent diarrhea. It dawned on me that my sweet cat really was seriously ill. The research I did on IBD suggested that if I couldn't get it under control, Duke might well succumb to intestinal lymphoma or, at least, be sentenced to a lifetime of feeling lousy. Once he was sufficiently stabilized and back home, I consulted a homeopathic vet who treated Duke for vaccinosis and, despite my intense trepidation, tried making some of the complicated raw diets I'd read about in my holistic care books. These diets included grains and vegetables. Some of the recipes made him vomit. All of them were complicated and I was overwhelmed with and worried by contradictory guidance about supplements. I was pretty close to giving up on this madcap "raw idea" altogether.

With help and patient guidance from a handful of (wonderful) people, including Michelle Bernard, I learned of an elegantly simple, raw, grainless diet that was based on re-creating the nutritional profile of a cat's natural prey. The common sense in this was inescapable, but I had serious reservations. After all, if the answer was *that* simple, *surely* vets would know it and tell everyone with an IBD cat to switch their cats to this diet. Right? Wrong.

I took three weeks to fully transition him and our other cat to the raw diet. I held my breath waiting for them both to keel over from eating food that didn't have that reassuring "100 percent nutritionally complete" label. They didn't keel over. Within 24 hours of eating nothing but the raw diet, all of Duke's symptoms disappeared. Completely.

It's been 26 months since he's been on the raw diet and 26 months since Duke has produced anything but perfect "tootsie-roll" stools. In those first days on raw, Duke seemed just as shocked at what was coming out his back end as I was. Today, he is a different, happier cat. He looks terrific and no longer sleeps in the crouched position that came from his always feeling like his insides were turning against him.

Duke is well, for the first time in his life, and it's the raw diet that did it. The answer, as it turns out, really was that simple."

Anne Jablonski

About seven years ago I took in a stray gold and black shorthaired kitten. He was covered in grease and very small for his age, which we guessed to be about two months old. Over the course of the next several years, Kit had numerous health issues, including periodic, severe urinary tract infections, and flare-ups of stomatitis (lesions in his mouth). To control the lesions, Kit would receive steroid shots about every 4-5 months.

After the last two shots that Kit received, he developed a severe upper respiratory infection. He was placed on antibiotics, primarily Baytril and antihistamines. I had to separate him from my other four cats for up to six weeks each time. During one of his vet visits, a heart murmur was detected. He had X-rays, an EKG and finally an ultrasound. He was diagnosed with feline hypertrophic cardiomyopathy (HCM), however he was unable to take the prescribed medication as it caused vomiting every day.

In July of 2002, I changed Kit to a raw diet. Over the course of the next few weeks, Kit lost weight. He needed to lose some weight, but this weight loss appeared to be excessive. So we went back to the vet. Kit had actually only lost about a quarter of a pound rather than the two pounds he appeared to have lost. He was now cat shaped rather than sausage shaped. Kit had really just shed the excess fluids he had been retaining.

Since July, Kit has now maintained a stable weight of 12 pounds. At first, he had a lot of excess skin on his stomach, but over time that has gone away, in part because he is much more active. He no longer has trouble breathing. The excess fluids were causing his heart to work much harder, so this diet is a significant benefit to him. Since the transition to raw, Kit has not had a flare up of stomatitis, although it is too soon to assume that he will never have another problem with this. Finally, Kit has a check-up for his heart in March of 2003. Kit looks and feels so much better than his last appointment. I am anxious to see if his heart disease has slowed (or reversed?!) In any case, the quality of his life has improved dramatically.

Susan Hiers

"We raise both Bengals and Classic Siamese, having approximately 10-18 resident cats at any time, not counting kittens. One of our F2 Bengals came to us after a severe allergic reaction to Albon, during which she made massive sores from scratching, especially at the injection site, lost 2/3 of her coat. When we got her, it appeared her problems were over from the reaction. NOT!!! Even after 2 months of steroids, antibiotics, etc., she was still pulling hair something terrible. You could feel scabs, her coat was dull, she had lost all kinds of weight, gotten pyometriosis, Giardia and Cryptosporidium, you name it, she had it! She had it over that period of time due to her immune system being out of whack because of the cortisones, steroids, antibiotics, etc she had been given to stop the itching, heal the sore, and rid her of the internal parasites. She was one miserable looking and feeling cat, and didn't want to be touched by anyone!!

We tried every type of canned and processed food on the market, including some mail-order foods; nothing helped her. On a whim, after sitting as a lurker on a couple of raw food cat lists and doing a lot of reading on processed cats foods, I decided to take the leap and try the raw food, it couldn't hurt, right? I went to 2 different health food stores, bought all kinds of ingredients included on the shopping lists from a couple of different raw feeding sites, and also got natural chicken, eggs, etc, and proceeded to make my first batch! What a learning experience! My cats are used to me cooking chicken for them, but I couldn't cut up the raw chicken and give it to them fast enough! We ended up having to close them all out of the kitchen, they wouldn't leave me or the chicken I was trying to cut up and grind alone! Several hours later, I finally had the first batch finished, ground bones and all. This was all on a Kitchen Aid mixer with the grinder attachment, and it didn't really like doing the bones, it was a very slow process.

We let all the cats back into the kitchen, and Sweetie, about 7 months old, went crazy over this food, along with most of my other Bengals and Siamese. We went through almost half of the batch in about 10 minutes. Within a week we started seeing a big difference in her actions, not as much over-grooming or itching, and the coat was starting to shine.

Two weeks later, most of the scabs were gone and she had fuzz coming in.

A month later, no sores, no bald spots, and an extremely glittered coat was showing. Made a tremendous difference in her appearance, behavior, and outlook on life. She still tends to overgroom slightly, but doesn't pull the hair or make sores now, and won't touch kibble or canned food. If I run out of raw, I go buy a chicken breast, thigh, whatever to give her until I can get some more ground as she will starve rather than eat canned, including Felidae and Wellness!!

Needless to say, I went out and bought a much better grinder after see these results and have made my own food since then! This way I know what my cats are eating, and when necessary, I add extras to the mix for nursing moms, kittens, and convalescing cats. The nursing moms especially crave the mix, they seem to know it is good for their milk production and the high protein seems to help them a lot.

We now know another good thing about the raw is my neutered Siamese had quite a primordial pouch starting. Since going raw, that is all but gone. All the cats are at healthy weights, no one is over or under weight and the coats are fabulous! So shiny and luxurious it's hard to believe.

We definitely believe in the feeding raw diets to our cats. Please visit our cattery websites (www.mewagecattery.com for our Bengals, and www.thatsixtyscattery.com for the Siamese) and look at the pictures of truly healthy cats, fed raw chicken, turkey, and occasionally rabbit. I work full time outside the home, and use one day of each weekend just to grind food. It is nothing for me to grind up 6 whole chickens, or 2 whole turkeys for the next 2 weeks worth of food. It is well worth the extra time and effort it takes, but the cats are healthy and we don't have stomach problems such as we were seeing on the canned food.

I recently was talking to a Bengal breeder in Canada and mentioned feeding raw. She has a cat that she had taken off the raw food due to time constraints and the cat now has fur missing etc. Since hearing our story of Sweetie, she has decided to start the raw again, especially for this one cat."

Pam Sechrest

"When I got my cat George from the shelter, he was only 6 weeks old, and had an upper respiratory infection. I took him to the vet a week later, who said that this is normal for shelter cats, and that it should go away on its own within a week or so. After a couple of weeks, he was still runny nosed and gummy eyed and sneezing every few minutes, so I took him back to the vet. The vet looked at George, took his temperature and said that he must still be having a problem with the upper respiratory infection, but it wasn't bad and that George was getting better, and not to worry about it.

About 3 weeks after that, George still wasn't better, so I took him back again. This time, the vet suggested that George might be allergic to something, but since it wasn't too bad, to still not worry about it. At this point, I was fed up with having a runny nosed, gummy eyed cat that sneezed snot all over my apartment, so I started doing some research, found out about raw food, and started George on the diet from the Blakkatz website.

It was a fairly smooth transition once I took all the dry food out of the house, and a few days after going completely raw, I noticed a marked improvement in George's sneezing and another week or so after that, he was all cleared up...no runny nose, no gummy eyes, very little sneezing. Now, how do I know that this is because of feeding raw? George went missing for a few days, and the person who found him was feeding commercial food. When I got him back, he was sneezing his head off again! After a couple of days back on raw, he was fine.

My vet was not especially thrilled when I told him I was feeding George raw food, he was very concerned that he would get salmonella poisoning, or wouldn't be getting all the nutrition he needs, even after I showed him the recipe I was following. Over a year later, and the vet says that George is one of the healthiest cats he sees. He is not over- or underweight, and has not had any problems since going on raw."

Laura Loignon

"I did not notice Kitty had diarrhea until I converted her from an indoor/outdoor cat to a solely indoor cat. She did not use the litter box in the house when she was allowed outside. For all I know, she could have been having problems with diarrhea for years before I knew there was a problem.

When I took her to the vet for her annual shots, I mentioned the diarrhea. We tried every type of food under the sun. Nothing worked so the vet put her on antibiotics for two weeks. Suddenly she started forming stool. Unfortunately, as soon as she came off the antibiotics, the diarrhea came back. At one point, the vet suggested she may have to stay on antibiotics for the rest of her life. When we tried Hill's d/d prescription food, she had formed stools, but they were skinny and dry. She began to loss weight at an alarming rate.

In 1999, I had a blood panel done on Kitty and discovered her liver values were elevated. I switched her to a different prescription food, this one for liver problems. The diarrhea came back. I changed to a holistic veterinarian who carried a line of frozen raw pet food. Because I am a vegetarian, the thought of raw meat made my stomach turn. Because the prescription food was not working, I decided to try the raw food.

After switching to raw food for one meal, Kitty's stools were perfect. There was noticeable weight gain within a week's time. After a few months on the raw food I was buying from my veterinarian, I switched to a completely homemade raw diet. While the food I was buying from the veterinarian made a difference in Kitty's stool, she did not like the vegetables and was still losing weight. The food I was making contained no vegetables which made Kitty very happy. She ate well and the weight gain continued.

I switched all my cats and my dog to a homemade raw diet.

In December of 2000, Kitty started vomiting. Tests revealed a mass in her stomach. As with many IBD cases, Kitty had lymphoma. Before I could make the decision whether to try chemo or steroids, Kitty took a turn for the worst, and on January 4, 2001 I put her to sleep. Even though Kitty's story had a bad ending, I learned valuable lessons. If I had known she had IBD, I would not have continued to give her annual vaccinations. I know now that a properly prepared raw food diet is far superior to any commercial food, prescription or otherwise. I now use a holistic veterinarian who does not look at the symptoms as problems, but as clues to what the problem really is. I formed the IBD list at Yahoo Groups in order to share my knowledge with other people with IBD cats. When Kitty was first diagnosed, there was no such list. Today the IBD list has over 700 members and continues to grow."

Lee Ellis

"My family and I were looking to purchase a Siamese kitten to join our family. After looking many places we were excited to locate a cattery in the same state we were in. This beautiful kitten seemed to have problems from the start. I thought maybe he was having problems adjusting to his new family, but the diarrhea continued on too long. I took Elijah to the vet for a check up. He did have fever due to inflammation of the colon. He was prescribed antibiotics and put on prescription Feline i/d. A week later after the meds Elijah never really stopped with the diarrhea. It just got a little better and then progressively worse again. I would wake up to find him covered from head to toe with diarrhea. It is like he could not control himself and would sleep and roll all in it. What a mess! Kittens hate baths I had always heard, but I did find out the hard way. Elijah hated his baths in the kitchen sink.

We were averaging about a visit a month to the vet for fecal exams, check ups, prescription antibiotics and prescription food. Our vet was puzzled by Elijah's doing ok on the antibiotics, but once he was through with them he would get worse again. He decided after two more trips that Elijah had a sensitive colon and would need to be on prescription food for the rest of his life. I was told he probably had IBD and would have to stay on this food indefinitely. Even though Elijah still had diarrhea on this food, but not near as bad as he did on Fancy Feast and Royal Canin dry. This seemed to be a temporary answer, but one I was not satisfied with. Why couldn't Elijah be a normal kitty that we could cuddle and love without getting poop all over us? More importantly, I wanted him healthy and happy. I couldn't understand why the vet thought it was ok for him to have diarrhea on the prescription food, as long as it wasn't severe as it had once been.

After searching for remedies or anything that might improve Elijah. I found a group on the Internet dedicated to IBD cats. They were feeding their kitty's raw diets and shared all their experiences. Their cats had no diarrhea on this diet. I wanted to try everything but this. I did try many different things that seemed to make Elijah worse again. I was ready to take him back to the vet for more antibiotics. I thought he could not live like this for very much longer. So I made up a batch of this raw chicken, liver, etc. I could not believe how Elijah took to it. He loved it and gobbled it up as fast as I could put it on his plate. After one day this kitty had no more diarrhea. I was used to scooping at least 15 times a day out of his litter box. I can happily say we only have one firm poop a day now. I have a happy eight-month-old kitten that has come to life and we are enjoying his new personality. I am so thankful that I found out about the benefits of a raw diet. It has totally changed our life."

Janna Jerry

In the summer of 1999, I brought home a blue Somali named Maggie. She was about a year and half old, and we just seemed to click. She did, however, have a health issue. From the time that Maggie was spayed, she had a problem with diarrhea. I took her to my allopathic vet, who ran blood work to help determine what was causing this, or at least to rule out what was not. The analysis did not identify a specific health issue, so the vet felt that it might either be inflammatory bowel disease (IBD) or perhaps a food allergy. As the tests for IBD can be very stressful as well as costly, she felt we should treat for IBD and see how Maggie responds.

Over the course of the next three years, Maggie was on various medications, but primarily on prednisolone and metronidazole with periodic steroid injections. We tried various diets, looking for a novel protein source or low allergen diet in case the issue was a food intolerance. During the course of these three years, we tried every approach that my vet was knowledgeable about as well as some supplements that were recommended by others who have cats with health issues. None of these medications, supplements or diets were effective. Maggie had gone from seven and a half pounds down to five pounds. Her coat was greasy and matted and emitted a foul odor. I had to bathe her every other week. She was frequently in pain.

In May of 2002, I began taking Maggie to a holistic vet and we tried acupuncture treatments and some other supplements. She went from five pounds to five and a half pounds and seemed to be improving a bit, but very slowly. In early July of 2002, she had an annual exam with a different vet from our regular clinic. He did not check her ears or her teeth, but did give her a three-year rabies vaccination and a steroid shot. I did not realize at the time that a vaccination should not be given to a sick animal and that a steroid shot and vaccination would work against each other. Maggie got worse and I decided I needed to take matters into my own hands. So I began my research by looking for as much information as I could find about feline IBD. I found a website for those who have cats with IBD, and to my surprise about 90 percent of the posts were about diet and nutrition. After two weeks of intense research I decided to try a raw diet.

After four weeks on a raw diet, Maggie no longer had diarrhea. This was the first time in over three years that she's had a formed stool. She slowly gained back her weight and I was able to wean her off the prescription drugs she was taking. She had more energy and was playful and once again willing to defend "her" territory. Her coat was cleaner, fuller and softer and I no longer had to bathe her.

Susan Hiers

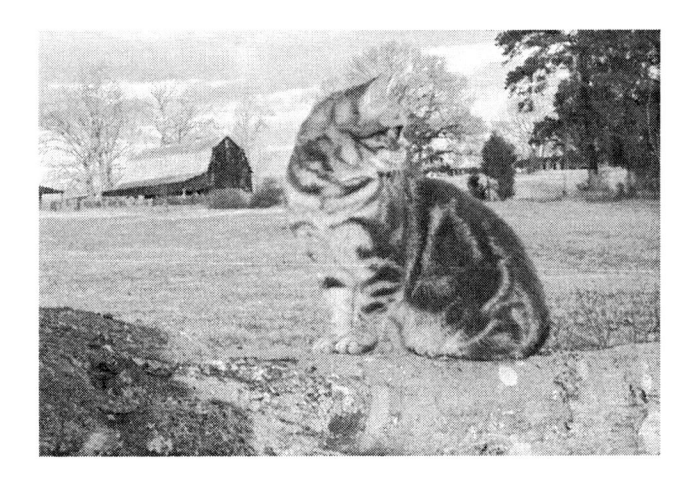

Chapter 20 – Homeopathy

Homeopathy is a wonderful healing art that was discovered by Samuel Hahnemann (1755-1843) in the late 1700s while he was working as a translator. Hahnemann was a medical doctor and a chemist. Disenchanted by medicine at the time, he stopped practicing medicine and was translating medical texts to support himself and his family. While translating a book by a physiologist named William Cullen, Hahnemann disputed the author's explanation of how Peruvian bark (cinchona) cured malaria. He did something that was unheard of in his time – he took several doses of Peruvian bark that caused him to develop fever, chills and other symptoms similar to malaria.[101]

Similia Similibus Curentur – "Like Cures Like." Any substance which can produce a totality of symptoms in a healthy human being can cure that totality of symptoms in a sick human being.[102]

Hahnemann spent the rest of his life developing the healing art he coined "homeopathy" from the Greek words *homoios* meaning "similar" and *pathos* meaning suffering. Homeopathy recognizes the symptoms evidenced by any living being as evidence of the disease and it is these symptoms *taken in their totality* that will guide the physician to the correct medicine to cure the patient, not just the disease. The totality of the symptoms is an expression of the essence of the disease. [103]

Homeopathy works on a dynamic or energetic level. Hahnemann used the term "vital force" to describe the spirit-like energy force that maintains the life of the individual. Without the vital force, the body dies.[104] When the vital force is in a state of balance, health exists. A cat (or any living creature) with a strong vital force (not to be confused with immune system because they are two different things) will be able to withstand exposure to certain disease stimulants with little disruption. One with a weak vital force, however, will be pushed to a state of imbalance with the slightest provocation.

This may be a difficult concept to understand, but a cat with a strong vital force will express a lot of symptoms when ill (or in a state of imbalance). For example, he may have a high fever and lots of discharge if sick with an upper respiratory infection. A cat with a weak vital force will express few symptoms and they will often be very weak, like a chronic low-grade fever. Obviously, it is much easier treating a cat with a strong vital force because there are often a lot of symptoms to go by.

A properly prescribed homeopathic remedy will work with the cat's vital force to remove the disease state. Treating a cat in this manner works to improve the vital force and because the symptoms are not suppressed the cat's overall immune system is strengthened as well.

The immune system is an internal force consisting of various components like the skin, nose, mouth, thymus, spleen and lymph system, designed to keep infections organisms out and destroying the ones that get in. If your cat has a competent immune system, he will be able to deal with infectious organisms without needing medicine of any kind. A kitten is born with a weak or undeveloped immune system. As the kitten matures and his immune system is challenged, preferably in a natural manner instead of by using vaccines, he develops natural immunity.

Conventional medicine views symptoms as something that must be crushed, wiped out, and stopped. If a cat has a runny nose or runny eyes, an antihistamine or antibiotic is prescribed; if diarrhea or vomiting is the symptom, anti-diarrhea or anti-vomiting medicine is given; for any inflammation or suspected inflammation occurs, steroids (an anti-inflammatory) are used. With conventional medicine, each symptom is treated using an opposing (or anti) medicine and the symptoms are suppressed, which does not cure the disease and may cause harm to the cat.

Conventional doctors blame disease on pathogens like germs, bacteria or a virus. They do blood tests, cultures or stool tests to find the culprit then they give the disease a name. Homeopathy does not name diseases, the practitioner makes note of symptoms no matter how minor or unusual and it is the symptoms that lead to a cure. People will often ask me what remedy is good for this disease or that disease? There is never one particular remedy for a disease condition. For example, a cat with inflammatory bowel disease would receive a remedy based on the *symptoms* the cat was expressing, not the inflammatory bowel *disease*. There are many different remedies for a disease like inflammatory bowel disease – it all depends on the symptoms.

A breeder taking a litter of kittens suffering from an upper respiratory infection into a conventional veterinarian's office would probably receive the same drug or drugs for all of the kittens. Even if one of the kittens in the litter were not showing symptoms, that kitten would probably receive the same medicine as the sick kittens, "just in case."

The same kittens taken to see a homeopath would quite possibly receive a different remedy, based on that kitten's *totality* of symptoms or *symptom picture*. The homeopathic remedy prescribed to each individual kitten would take into account the kitten's particular personality, temperature preference, and food preference as well as the symptoms attributed to the upper respiratory infection. If one of the kittens had soft stool, passed gas or had a cough, in addition to the eye and nose symptoms that would be taken into account. Nothing about that kitten would be ignored or thought of as not part of the symptom picture or disturbance. The whole kitten is treated – *not just the disease*. If there was a kitten in the litter that was not showing symptoms, he would not receive a remedy, "just in case."

A conventional veterinarian seeing a kitten with upper respiratory symptoms and runny stool would probably culture the kitten's mucus and stool to define what organism or organisms caused the illness. The upper respiratory symptoms would be treated with one drug and the runny stool with another. Both drugs would be prescribed in an effort to stop the symptoms. Both drugs would probably have their residual side effects as well. The antibiotic would destroy the healthy bacteria in the kitten's system and if the kitten had runny stool because of some toxin in the kitten's food, the toxin would not be expelled from the kitten's body as quickly as it should be because the anti-diarrhea medicine would prevent diarrhea.

> *The physician's highest calling, his **only** calling, is to make sick people healthy – to heal, as it is termed.*
> *– Samuel Hahnemann*

The above paragraph contained in Hahnemann's *Organon of Medicine* is the first "rule" of homeopathy. Stop and think here. With the exception of some surgeries, emergency medicine, and antibiotics in the case of some life-threatening bacterial infections, does conventional veterinary medicine ever make sick animals healthy? Or does it merely suppress the symptoms (usually temporarily) or manage the disease?

Does conventional veterinary medicine even know what *healthy* is? Conventional veterinarians are taught what disease is and how to try to cure it with drugs. If an animal may be exposed to a virus (or even if they may not be exposed), you vaccinate to prevent the animal from getting the virus, or you treat the virus with a drug that will make the symptoms go away. If some part of the animal is causing a problem, like, for example impacted anal glands, you remove the offending anal glands. If there is inflammation, you make it go away with steroids. A conventional veterinarian rarely gets to the root of the problem or tries to figure out *why* the problem is occurring. He looks at the symptoms and prescribes a drug or therapy that will stop the symptoms.

On the other side of the coin, does conventional veterinary medicine really know what a *sick* cat is? Is the cat that runs under the bed whenever company arrives or is licking himself raw considered sick? The cat with tissue damage is surely sick, but what about the one that bites if he is petted for too long? What most conventional veterinarians do not understand is that the cat that is sucking its tail or licking herself raw *is* sick and tissue damage is on its way. If they could find a way to treat the cat now with something that is not going to suppress the symptoms *before* the tissue damage occurs, they would be ahead of the game.

Getting to the root of the problem would never happen during a 15-minute office visit. A typical initial appointment with a homeopath may take as long as an hour or two. Do not be scared away by the initial consultation fee for a homeopath. Multiply a conventional veterinarian's office visit fee by four and see what it comes to. The appointment with a homeopath does not end with the consultation. After it is over, the homeopath begins research to find the right remedy for your cat.

In several places throughout this book I say that I believe commercial cat food causes various feline ailments such as feline urinary tract disease, inflammatory bowel disease, and several others, but that is not quite true. Some cats live their entire lives on cheap store brand dry cat food without ever showing symptoms of disease. They die in their sleep at a ripe old age. There are some people who work at extremely stressful jobs, eat fast food almost every day, get little sleep, smoke and drink and never get sick. These scenarios are not terribly common anymore. That cat that lived to a ripe old age on cheap food probably lived outside, hunted to supplement the dry food and may not have been vaccinated on an annual basis. Cats do not live that way these days. They are indoor couch potatoes who are taken to the veterinarian for medicine for every sneeze or runny eye, vaccinated every year, and fed processed food.

It is the underlying susceptibility or sensitivity to a particular disease process that allows the cat to get sick. Susceptibility to particular diseases passes through the generations. No matter what conventional veterinary reports say, cats are *not* getting healthier. They are succumbing to serious chronic disease and dying at young ages. Even if they live to old age, what is the quality of their life if they have a chronic disease and receive daily medicine, fluids, and eat a prescription diet? I am not concerned with a 16-year-old cat with failing kidneys. Organs fail with old age – that is normal. I am concerned with an 8-year-old cat that dies from chronic renal failure. There is something wrong with that picture.

> *"My barn having burned to the ground,*
> *I can now see the moon."*
> *-- Zen haiku*

Every single symptom your cat exhibits is there for a reason – it is an express of the disease state your cat is suffering from. It is only by careful observation of these symptoms that you can successfully cure your cat. Sneezing, runny eyes, coughing and fever are good signs of immune response on the part of your cat – especially if it is an acute illness like an upper respiratory infection. A cat that spends weeks or months with a little bit of discharge and a low-grade fever is not showing a strong immune response. Diarrhea and vomiting are an attempt to move the toxin quickly through the system to prevent damage to the vital organs. The body heals through excretions – do not stop this normal process. Stopping these symptoms is done to the detriment of the cat.

Of course you should contact a veterinarian, preferably a holistic veterinarian, if any symptom, especially a high fever, vomiting or diarrhea, persists for longer that a few days.

Miasms

"Miasm" was a term coined by Samuel Hahnemann to explain an underlying tendency to get sick. In lay terms, a miasm is a weakness or susceptibility that leads to disease or illness, often passing through the generations, although not all miasms are inherited. Some miasms are created by drug toxicity or faulty treatment (such as use of steroids) and those caused by infectious miasms (natural diseases). These "created" miasms can also pass through generations.

Today, manmade toxins, such as those contained in the environment and even in commercial pet food, need to be included into causes of disease as well as vaccine miasms that are becoming increasingly common in cats. Chronic illnesses that include several factors of causation, stress, natural diseases (infections), drugs, toxins and vaccines, are extremely difficult to cure, even with homeopathy. It needs to be done by an experienced homeopath and it takes a great deal of patience and observation skills on the part of the caregiver.

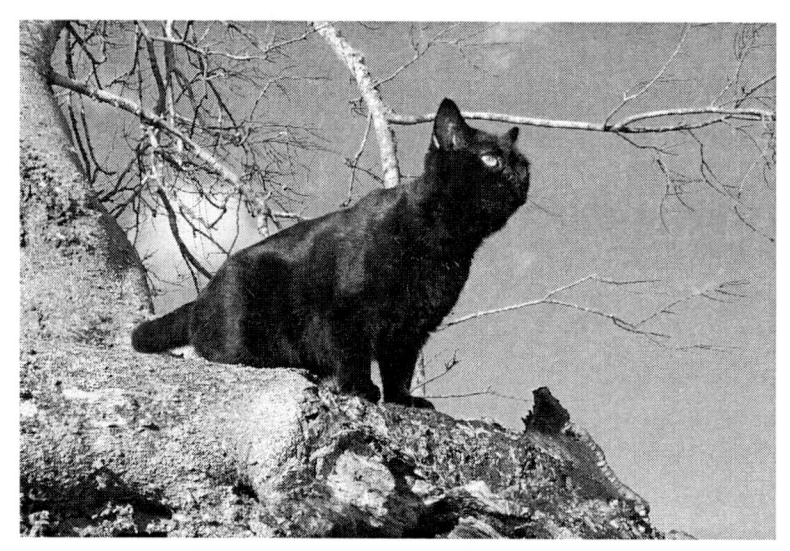

What you need to remember is disease or illness does not necessarily come from viruses or bacteria, it comes from *within* the cat. It is an *underlying susceptibility*

to that particular influence. Bacteria and viruses are opportunistic; they go for unhealthy or susceptible creatures.

The disease and the creature are linked on an energy level. A miasm is a weakness in the creature's vital force that allows an opening to form, letting in the disease.

How do homeopathic remedies work?

In health, your cat goes about his business and everything is great – he is in a state of equilibrium. Then one day, something, whether it is a virus, bacteria, trauma, or toxin, attempts to push your cat's vital force off balance. Your cat will start to show symptoms of disease – his vital force needs help righting itself. The vital force is unable to cure itself – it needs help.

You can do one of two things – you can take your cat to a conventional veterinarian who will examine your cat, maybe perform laboratory tests and give your cat something that is going to make the symptoms go away; *or* you can take the cat to your homeopath, tell him the symptoms your cat is exhibiting and the homeopath will prescribe a homeopathic remedy that can cause symptoms very similar to those your sick cat is exhibiting.

Remember, the homeopathic remedy you give your cat is working on an energy level, just like the vital force is. You cannot see the vital force working – you can only see the symptoms. The energy of the homeopathic remedy (think of it as an artificial disease) is going to be very similar in action to the energy (or the natural disease) that caused the disturbance in your cat, but it is somewhat stronger. The artificial disease replaces the natural disease and then fades and the vital force takes over again. The difference between treating a cat with homeopathy compared to conventional treatment is with homeopathy the disease state is removed, not the symptoms. When the disease state is removed, the symptoms go along with it.

Sometimes a homeopathic remedy will work quickly. Usually this occurs in an acute case – something that comes on suddenly, often violently, like a sudden fever, vomiting or diarrhea. An acute disease or disorder should resolve quickly with a properly chosen homeopathic remedy. If in an acute disease a remedy does not work rapidly, you have the option of trying a different remedy. With a chronic condition, something that comes on slowly, homeopathy is probably not going work as quickly as conventional medicine. This is where so many people leave homeopathy and go back to conventional medicine. They do not want to wait for a cure. Patience is probably the hardest thing to learn about homeopathy. Caregivers do not want to sit around and watch their cat scratch, ooze mucus or have diarrhea.

> *"When clouds form in the skies we know that rain will follow but we must not wait for it. Nothing will be achieved by attempting to interfere with the future before the time is ripe. Patience is needed."*
> — *I Ching*

Choosing a competent homeopath is very important. It takes many years of study and practice to become good at prescribing. Improper homeopathic treatment of a case can sometimes cause more damage than conventional medicine because homeopathy works on a deeper (energetic) level than conventional medicine.

I have seen some miraculous cures in my cats by using homeopathy, but rarely does it happen overnight. I see some parallels between Buddhism and homeopathy. In Buddhism suffering is thought of as opportunity. If you can get through the suffering and be aware throughout the process you grow. Everything changes and even if it seems like your cat has suffered for months during homeopathic treatment, it will change, I promise you that. In homeopathy, sometimes the cat will have to suffer a bit longer before a remedy works. It may take several remedies before you see a cure. Covering up the suffering as conventional medicine does with its antibiotics and steroids is not curing the condition. It is sweeping it under the rug. Ultimately, the symptoms will come back, sometimes worse than they were to begin with. There are no quick fixes or magic bullets in life.

When I first discovered homeopathy I wanted to cure the World with this wonderful medicine. I started fostering cats, bringing in more than I could handle at the time. Almost as soon as I acquired a cat I would schedule a homeopathic consultation. While I do not think I ever caused harm to a cat, I probably wasted a lot of money in homeopathic treatment. Usually, the cats that were treated were not exhibiting clear symptoms. You cannot really learn about a cat when you have only known her for a month or two. Without a clear-cut symptom picture, it is difficult to find the right remedy. Again, patience is the key. While you can learn about the cat's temperament and preferences on a day-to-day basis, often you need to wait for something to cause the cat's vital force to act. Then you have symptoms to work with. A properly chosen homeopathic remedy used during an acute disease will often cause the animal to exhibit new symptoms that will lead you to a long-term remedy. This is known as the cat's "constitutional remedy." The acute disease will help you to discover where the cat's sensitivities lie, what underlying susceptibilities he has. Wait and watch.

"You can do foolish things, but do them with enthusiasm"
— *Colette*

Because I use homeopathy to treat illnesses in my cats, I have to be extremely diligent and observant in their care. I have to keep my numbers down. There is no way I can care for or treat a large number of cats using these methods. When I had more cats than could comfortably live in the environment I provided, they got sick more often. Cats do not deal well with overcrowding or stress. They seem to be more sensitive to stress than other animals. Cats are highly spiritual creatures and homeopathy works really well with them, but I have to walk a fine line with their care. There are obstacles to cure: poor quality diet, bad hygiene, stress and vaccination. I do not think I would be as successful using homeopathy if they were fed a commercial diet, vaccinated every year and lived in cages or overcrowded conditions. Homeopathy is probably not going to help a person that gets sick after working 60 hours a week at a high stress job, eating a steady diet of fast food and sleeping four hours a night. A cat living in crowded conditions without exposure to sun and fresh air, eating meat flavored cereal and that is vaccinated every year is probably not going to respond to homeopathy either.

Where do homeopathic remedies come from?

Research on the action of homeopathic remedies, called "provings," are conducted using healthy humans and in some instances by studying accidental poisonings. The term "proving" comes from the German word, *prüfen* meaning to test. Homeopathic remedies are tested on healthy humans. If there is no other reason to use homeopathy, use it because the medicine is not tested on animals. No laboratory animals suffer through horrible experiments to test homeopathic remedies before they are used on humans. Each subject involved in a proving is asked to keep detailed notes throughout the process. The information obtained from a proving is compiled in the Materia Medica then the information from the Materia Medica is indexed in the Repertory.

Homeopathic remedies are not given in their crude form. That is why very dangerous substances like deadly nightshade, arsenic and snake poisons can be used safety. Use of remedies in their crude form, even if given in very minute amounts or diluted caused illness or aggravations in Hahnemann's early patients. He wanted to be able to use the more poisonous materials like arsenic or mercury, but he was afraid to test such dangerous substances in order to discover their curative ability. Hahnemann experimented by diluting the substance many thousands of times. Much to his amazement, he discovered the more diluted the remedy, the more powerful and long acting it became. Homeopathic remedies are not simply diluted. Each dilution is vigorously shaken throughout the process (called "succussion"). This dilution and shaking makes the remedy stronger. Conventional potencies are so diluted that there are no detectable molecules of the original substances left. All that is left is the energy or essence of the substance. Homeopathy is an energy healing modality.

A 30c potency is a serial dilution of 1 to 100 made thirty times (10^{60}). A 30c potency is a relatively low potency, with 1M ($10^{2,000}$), 10M ($10^{20,000}$) and 50M ($10^{100,000}$) potencies being used in practice today. A 1M potency is far more powerful and long acting than the 30c potency. That is what those numbers (6c, 30c, 200c, 1M) mean on the side of a homeopathic remedy vial.

Do not let anyone tell you it is necessary for an aggravation to occur before your cat is cured. Aggravations are not necessary and should be avoided at all costs. A single homeopathic remedy should be given in the lowest potency necessary to cure the patient.

How to Find a Homeopathic Veterinarian

Back when I started using homeopathy with my cats the problem with using a homeopathic vet was finding one. There were not too many practicing homeopathic vets.

Today, it seems that everyone is jumping on the bandwagon. I am not surprised. It happened with raw diet and natural medicine (herbs and supplements). Do an Internet search for raw diet, BARF (an acronym for "bones and raw food" or "biologically appropriate food"), or natural health for animals and you will find web page after web page selling products. All these combinations and concoctions are supposed all to help your dog or cat get over whatever ails them. Many of them are nothing more than empty promises of quick fixes and are no better than conventional medicine.

If you go looking for a natural remedy for a skin condition, you will find hundreds. Remedies, even if they are natural, can suppress just like conventional medicine.

There are seminars available for veterinarians to learn homeopathy. A conventionally trained veterinarian *cannot* become a homeopathic veterinarian after taking a few seminars on veterinary homeopathy. It does not happen that quickly. They have to change their whole manner of thinking to become good homeopaths. This process takes many years of careful study.

When looking for a homeopathic veterinarian, keep a few things in mind and ask questions. Interview the homeopathic veterinarian before you put your money down.

Look for a homeopathic veterinarian that practices 75-100 percent homeopathy. Nothing less will do. If the homeopathic veterinarian practices Chinese medicine, acupuncture and homeopathy, he is not specialized enough. He needs to focus close to 100 percent on homeopathy. A good place to start is on-line at The Academy of Veterinary Homeopathy, **http://www.theavh.org** or by telephone at 866-652-1590.

It is usually not a good idea to mix healing modalities. You probably should not use acupuncture and homeopathy at the same time. They both use energy to heal and may counteract each other. If you are using herbs and homeopathy and your cat improves, you will not know what actually worked, the homeopathy or the herbs. It is best to keep it simple and use one type of healing at a time. This does not mean you cannot make an herbal tea to bathe your cat's eyes and nose if he has a cold. Use of herbs on the surface is usually not going to confuse things. You should avoid giving herbs or even extra nutritional supplements orally while using homeopathy. It could confuse the symptom picture.

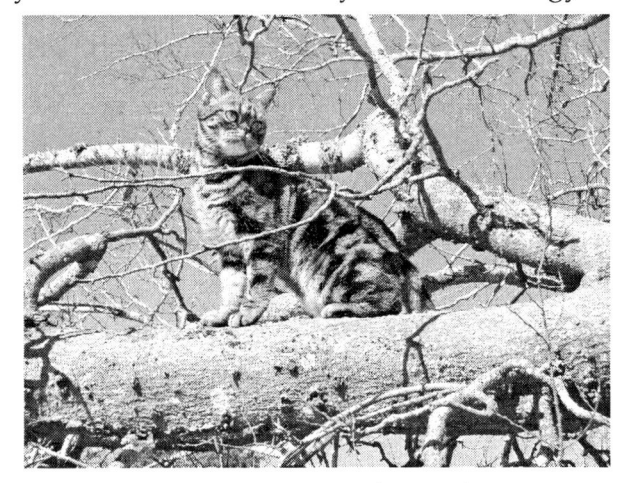

You do not have to go to the vet. If you can find one that meets the qualifications I have laid out in the following paragraphs in your own state, great! You may not be able to. Many homeopathic veterinarians do telephone consultations. Some states may have legislation pending preventing telephone consultations with out of state veterinarians. You may need to check into this. Prior to a telephone consultation, you can have your animal's records sent to the homeopathic vet. You should send a picture of your cat as well.

Find a homeopathic veterinarian that has been in practice for more than a few years and one that has taken human courses. For example the Devon School for Homeopathy offers a wonderful correspondence course. Many good homeopathic veterinarians have studied with human homeopaths. Homeopathy works the same for humans as it does for animals. It's the principles of homeopathy that are important, not what you are healing.

You will want to ask the homeopathic veterinarian if he or she believes aggravations are necessary. Although they may occur and should be very mild, aggravations are not necessary to heal. Ask the veterinarian if he has read the *Organon* and what edition he practices by (it should be the 5th or 6th edition). If the veterinarian has not read or does not know what the *Organon* is, he is not a homeopathic vet. Ask the veterinarian when he last read the entire *Organon*. The *Organon*, written by Samuel Hahnemann, is considered the "bible" of homeopathy. The *Organon* explains exactly how homeopathy should be practiced. A good practitioner reads the entire *Organon* at least once a year.

Keep in mind you will probably have to wait to get an appointment with a good homeopathic veterinarian. If you are thinking of using one, find one now and make the appointment so the veterinarian will have a record of you so that if you really need him in a crisis, he'll be available.

Finally, read up on homeopathy. Have some idea of how it works. If you question something, then ask the vet. Communication and observation are imperative when you are using homeopathy. You need to watch and make note of everything, no matter how minor. Keeping a journal is an excellent idea.

The most important thing you need to know is that homeopathy is not going to act immediately, or at least it shouldn't unless you are working with an acute case. It should work slowly. The slower the better – patience is the key.

Buying Homeopathic Remedies

You can buy homeopathic remedies individually at most health food stores. That can run into a lot of money if you are going to be using homeopathy on a regular basis. I have the Washington 30c kit that is a set of 50 remedies in 30c potency that costs about $80.00. This kit is worth its weight in gold. You can purchase this kit directly from Washington Homeopathy on-line at **http://www.homeopathyworks.com/** or by calling 1-800-336-1695. You can also purchase it from Homeopathy Overnight at **http://www.homeopathyovernight.com** or by calling 1-800-276-4223. Both Washington and Homeopathy Overnight carry single remedies. Natural Health Supply, on-line at **http://a2zhomeopathy.com/** or by telephone (888) 689-1608, carries LM remedies, amber bottles and vials suitable for preparing LM homeopathic remedies, as well as single remedies and kits. For more obscure remedies or nosodes, Hahnemann Pharmacy has just about any remedy you may need, **http://www.hahnemannlabs.com/** 1-888-427-6422

With whatever remedy you purchase, ask for the #20 pellets. The small #20 pellets are easier to administer to cats because it is more difficult for them to spit out the tiny pellets. If you have to use the larger pellets, it is usually best to crush them between two clean spoons and then administer the powder.

I almost always use the 30c potency in my cats. It seems to be the potency that works without causing aggravations. With the 30c, especially in an acute illness or disturbance, I can switch remedies after 12 to 24 hours if it does not work.

It's always best to err on the side of caution and use low potencies. Try to not to give remedies too frequently, give the remedy time to work. Patience and understanding of the principles of homeopathy are paramount.

How to Administer a Homeopathic Remedy

I love using homeopathy on my cats because it is so easy to administer remedies. I have a few cats that are notoriously difficult to pill. I could not imagine having to administer medicine once or twice a day to these cats! I am so glad I discovered homeopathy!

Homeopathic remedies should not be given within 30 minutes of your cat having food in his mouth. You should not mix homeopathic remedies with any food except milk or cream. If your cat likes milk or cream, you can dissolve a few pellets in a clean glass saucer of milk or cream. Let your cat drink the milk or cream. He does not drink all of it in order for the remedy to work.

If your cat will not drink milk or cream, pour a few pellets, no more than three or four, into the cap of the remedy vial. *Do not* touch the pellets, the oils in your skin can contaminate a remedy. Gently open the cat's mouth and toss the pellets in. If you are using a remedy that is in the larger pellets, you may need to crush them into a powder between two clean spoons. I have found cats spit out the larger pellets. If it is in a powder or the tiny pellets, they usually cannot spit them all out. Even if only one pellet got in the cat's mouth, that is all you need. If any drop on the floor, throw them away.

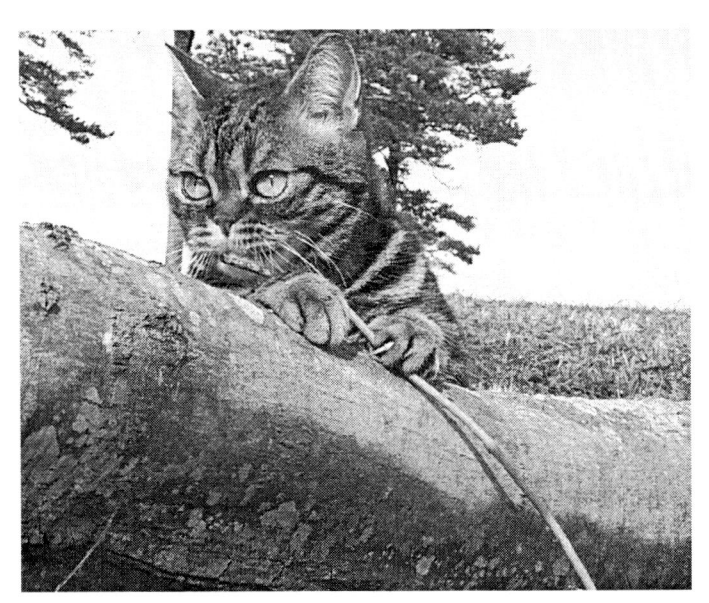

The same potency usually should not be administered more than once. If you need to give the remedy again, you should use the liquid method of dosing which changes the potency of the remedy ever so slightly. Dissolve one 30c pellet in a sterilized glass jar, or better yet, an amber vial (see resources) containing four ounces of spring water or distilled water. Put the cover on the jar strike it against the palm of your hand (brace your arm against your waist) five times. You can also put a towel on a countertop as a pad and strike the jar against the countertop. Draw off one spoonful of the water from the jar and stir it into a clean glass containing another four ounces of spring or distilled water. Stir the water in the second glass about ten times. Then give your cat a spoonful of the liquid from the second glass. You can use a glass eyedropper or stir the liquid into a bit of cream or milk. The liquid method of dosing is very gentle and often works better the dry dosing in sensitive subjects.

Now comes the hard part. You wait for the remedy to work and watch for new symptoms.

Chapter 21 – The Litter Box

Ranking right up there with giving their caregiver a hard time about switching to a raw diet are litter box problems. Out-of-litter-box experiences can drive many a caregiver to drink. It also results in many cats being surrendered to shelters or euthanized.

There is some thought that clay clumping litter may be ingested by your cat and contribute to blockage. This has not been verified, however, clay clumping litter is extremely dusty and that it is certainly not desirable for you or your cat to be inhaling clay dust. If your cat has excessively dry stools, try switching to a litter that is nonclumping and see if it makes a difference.

If at all possible, avoid clay litter in any form. Clay is mined from the earth and it is not biodegradable. It is dusty and dirty. If your cat insists on clay, use the cheapest brand you can find without added fragrance. A cat on a raw diet should not have smelly stool so you do not need added fragrance. Cats often object to strong smelling fragrances and it can cause allergic reactions in sensitive cats.

There are several natural clumping litters available. One is World's Best Cat Litter that is made from corn. Another brand is Swheatscoop made from wheat. Those people who use World's Best Cat Litter swear by it. They also swear when they go through the check out to buy it. World's Best Cat Litter is one of the most expensive natural cat litters on the market. Swheatscoop is more economical, but it has a tendency to stick to the sides of the litter box like cement. You may need to rent a jackhammer to get it off your litter box. One way to prevent this is to spray Pam or other nonstick spray on your litter box before filling it with Swheatscoop. While Swheatscoop costs less, you need to put more in the box than World's Best so the cost is probably comparable.

I do not like scooping litters because no matter how carefully you scoop, you never completely remove all of the soiled litter. The clumps break and some of the soiled litter falls back into the box. I have used Swheatscoop in the past and after it has been used for a few days it develops a distinctive sweet smell that is not terribly agreeable. The texture is certainly attractive to most cats as they prefer a sandy substance to eliminate in.

If you have a cat prone to constipation you may not want to use clumping litter. Your cat can ingest even the natural clumping litters and it may contribute to excessively dry stools. In fact, if you think your cat is constipated and you are using clumping litters, try changing the litter to see if it resolves.

Some carbo-junkie cats will eat the corn or wheat-based litter which defeats the purpose of a grain-free raw food diet.

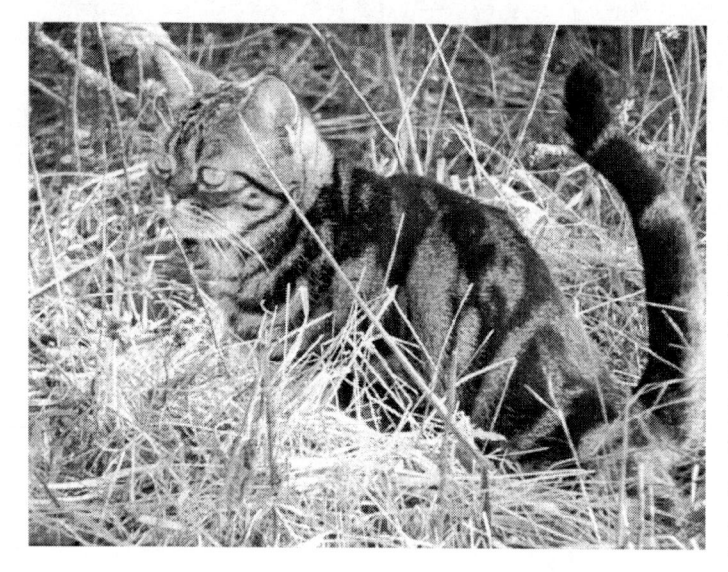

The next line of natural cat litter is the pellet type. The most common is Feline Pine. Other brands are Cat Country, Cat Works and Great Mews. All are made from environmentally friendly materials. Some cats object to pellet litter and quite frankly I do not blame them. It is hard on the feet and a foreign substance for cats to dig in. I know Feline Pine breaks down to a powder once it gets wet with urine. The manufacturer recommends removing the stool on a daily basis, leaving the rest of the litter behind until it is time to completely dump the box. That is leaving urine-soaked litter in the box – not the cleanest of methods. The combination of pine and urine scent in a box that is overdue for cleaning is very distasteful.

Carefresh Pet Bedding and Ecofresh Cat Litter are both made from paper and have the consistency of cornflakes.

I am sure I am missing a few brands, but this gives you an idea of the various brands of natural cat litter available.

More creative caregivers, especially those with multiple cats, go beyond the mainstream cat litter and use wood stove pellets (which is just like Feline Pine), chicken crumbles (like World's Best Cat Litter), corncob husks, alfalfa pellets, or beet pulp (like shredded paper).

If you use chicken crumbles, be sure you are buying an unmedicated brand. A lot of chicken food contains antibiotics that you do not want your cat consuming.

I have been using wood shavings for years. Wood shavings have all of the pros of a good litter, they are light, virtually dust-free and cheap. The only disadvantages are that they are so light the litter boxes need to be anchored to a nearby wall or they get tipped over when the cat jumps out of the box and they probably track more than some litters. The advantages outweigh the disadvantages in my household. I completely dump all of my litter boxes twice a day. If necessary, I spray them with a biodegradable cleaner, wipe them dry and refill them.

Keep the litter box simple. Do not invest money in automatic litter boxes. They do not work well and may frighten your cat so that he will never use another litter box again. You want to see what your cat is eliminating on a daily basis. Stool watching is a pastime you do not want to miss out on.

The covered litter boxes may be nice for the caregiver, but they were not created with the cat's best interests in mind. A large cat will need to stoop in an unnatural position in order to eliminate. A covered litter box makes for a great ambush if you have one cat in the household that likes to pick on another. With a covered litter box you may not notice that the litter box needs cleaning as quickly as you would with an uncovered one. You may not smell an odor coming from the box because it is covered and may have some form of filtration, but your cat certainly will smell it when he's using it. Think of a covered litter box like one of those porta-potties they have at fairs and some rest stops. Do you like using them? I certainly do not.

I use the giant-size litter boxes and have one litter box for every two cats in my household. If you have a cat that likes to stand upright while urinating midstream (some female cats like to do this), use one of those large plastic storage boxes you can get at any discount store.

The most important thing about a litter box is that it be kept in an out of the way place, away from your cat's food and water, and that it be kept clean. Cats are very clean creatures and appreciate a clean litter box.

If your cat is eliminating in an inappropriate place such as a plant, put bark chips or stones on top of the soil of the plant, or wrap aluminum foil around the top of the pot. Some cats like to eliminate behind or near potted plants. If this is the case with your cat, well then why not decorate the litter box area with some potted plants?

If your cat has discovered a corner that he would much rather use for a litter box, if possible, move the litter box there. Sometimes it is better to accommodate them when comes to location of a litter box. If you cannot move the litter box, put a small litter box in the location and use a few sheets of paper towel for litter. I do this when I have young kittens in the house. They often forget where the main litter boxes are and gravitate to the corners of the room to eliminate. I leave small litter boxes lined with paper towel in various corners throughout the house. Small kittens have a hard time getting into the large litter boxes so the small ones work well for them.

If you have a kitten that is having difficulty figuring out how to use the litter box, put a bit of soiled litter from another litter box in the one you want the kitten to use. Most get the idea right away. If not, confine the kitten to a small area with the one litter box within easy access. Sometimes if the kitten is kept in too large an area they have a hard time mastering the litter box.

Homeopathy can often correct elimination problems because they are usually psychological in nature. A cat will often eliminate inappropriately if they are angry with their caregiver. Feeding a raw diet certainly helps keep a cat on a good mental plane. If a cat is acting inappropriately while on commercial food I often suggest switching to raw to help temperament issues. A cat on a healthy diet is usually a happy cat.

There can certainly be health issues involved with a cat urinating inappropriately. If you have such a problem, a urinary tract infection or other disorder should be considered as a possible contributor, especially if the cat is urinating small amounts on a frequent basis.

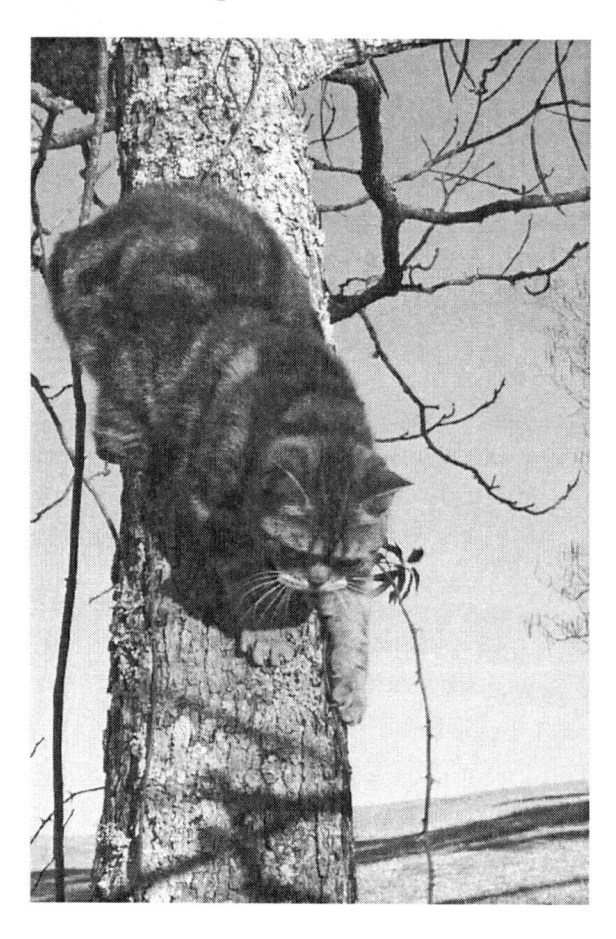

Chapter 22 – The Scratching Post

Cats need to keep their claws in good shape and a good scratch stretches the cat's muscles. Cats have to scratch and they like to climb. A good scratching post is as important as diet and the litter box.

I like the Felix brand scratching post. I have had mine for years and years and they are still in excellent condition. Felix is a small company in Washington State. It will take a few weeks to get your post, but they are well worth the wait. The telephone number for Felix is 1-206-547-0042. Order the 30 inch post which is approximately $50.00 including shipping and handling.

If there is a cat show in your area, there will probably be a scratching post vendor present. You can usually get a good scratching post at a cat show for a better price than you can in a pet store. Do not buy a post covered with carpet as it may encourage your cat to scratch on carpet. Stick with sisal rope or sisal fabric. To check for cat shows in your area, check the CFA web site at **http://www.cfainc.org** or the TICA web site at **http://www.tica.org.**

If you are handy and patient you can make your own scratching post covered with sisal rope. Sisal rope is available at most hardware stores.

I made a handmade scratching post out of a large tree branch nailed to a base partially wrapped in sisal rope. My cats also have a five-foot wooden stepladder wrapped in sisal rope. They love the ladder as you can see from the photo to the right. It can be hard to find a wooden stepladder these days though. You could make a regular ladder out of wood and wrap that with sisal rope.

Another brand that I have been told cats love is one made by Cosmic Catnip called the Alpine Scratcher. It is made from corrugated cardboard. I have a Turbo Scratcher — a round plastic toy with a ball in the track and a piece of corrugated cardboard in the middle to scratch on. Rooney in particular likes to scratch on this toy. Both of these toys are readily available on the Internet and at major pet supply chain stores like PetSmart.

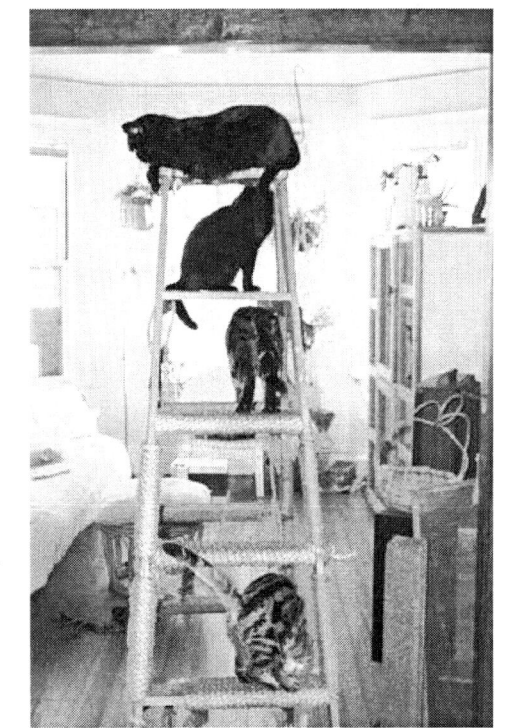

Chapter 23 - Vaccination

The following statement is from a very well respected veterinary book, Current Veterinary Therapy. The authors are veterinary immunologists Ronald Schultz (University of Wisconsin) and Tom Phillips (Scrips Research Institute).

> "A practice that was started many years ago and that lacks scientific validity or verification is annual revaccination. Almost without exception there is no immunologic requirement for annual revaccination. Immunity to viruses persists for years or for the life of the animal. ... Furthermore, revaccination with most viral vaccines fails to stimulate an anamnestic (secondary) response. ... The practice of annual vaccination in our opinion should be considered of questionable efficacy ..."

I am not going to say much on this topic because it could end up being another book and others have already said it much more eloquently. Conduct an Internet search for the first few words of the above quote and you will find web page after web page on the subject.

Donald Hamilton, DVM discusses vaccination in his book, *Homeopathy Care for Cats and Dogs*, as does Richard Pitcairn, DVM in *Natural Health for Dogs and Cats*. Catherine O'Driscoll wrote a whole book on the dangers of vaccination, *What Vets Don't Tell You About Vaccines*. There are numerous books geared towards humans and vaccine damage such as *A Shot in the Dark* by Harris Coulter, *What Your Doctor May Not Tell You About Children's Vaccinations* by Stephanie Cave, *Vaccinations 100 Years of Orthodox Research* by Viera Scheibner to name a few.

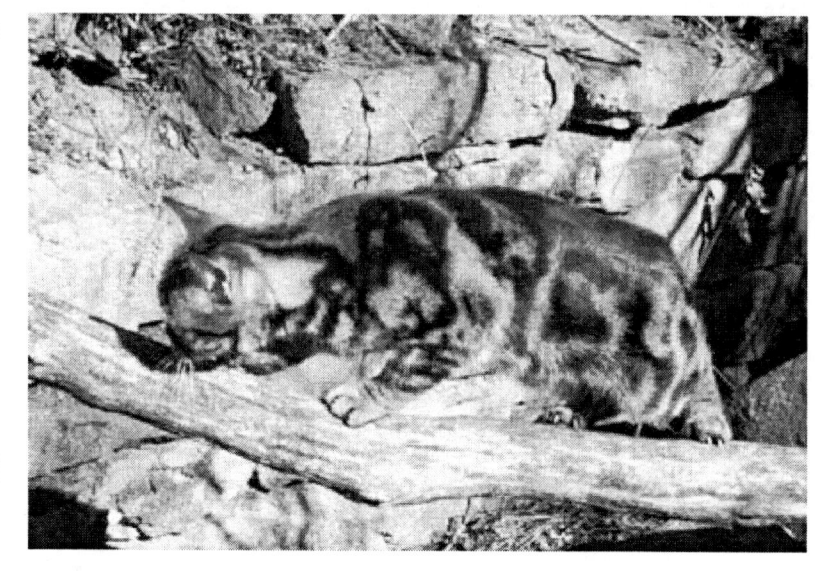

Except for rabies that is required by law, my cats have not been vaccinated for anything since 1993. My older cats were vaccinated as kittens. All of the cats that I breed have not been vaccinated for anything except rabies (because it is required by law). After the research I have conducted over the years, I am more afraid of the vaccine than I am of the disease the vaccine is supposed to prevent against it. Tangle, who is shown in several photographs throughout this book, is second generation unvaccinated.

The introduction of several manmade viruses into a cat's blood stream via an injection is an unnatural way for a cat to encounter a virus. Most viruses would enter the mucous membranes (the nose and mouth) where the cat's first line of defense would begin. If the virus (and it's rarely more than just one virus) is injected into the blood stream, the immune system of the cat is caught off guard without an opportunity to begin a normal defense strategy. The cat is doing just fine and then all of a sudden three or more viruses have invaded its blood stream. No wonder autoimmune diseases are so common in cats. The intra-nasal vaccines are a more natural method of introducing a virus, but the intra-nasals tend to not be as effective as the injected vaccines. The intra nasals are also modified live viruses that can cause the disease. Using a modified live panleukopenia virus vaccine could cause panleukopenia. Killed vaccines have their own inherent dangers. I believe the only safe form of vaccination is no vaccination.

Chris Kurz, who has a Ph.D in physics and has been practicing homeopathy for many years, has a great analogy for the harm in annual vaccination:

> "On the drive to work I started to think about homeopathy and vaccination. For somebody not familiar with homeopathy it is tempting to put those two in the same mental drawer and 'explain' one with the other. Here is my personal metaphor that I use to point out the important difference between the two to somebody who doesn't know much about homeopathy:
>
> Picture your body as a mansion containing many valuable things which need to be protected from burglars. The owner of the mansion (i.e. you) has hired security guards to do the job.
>
> Now, one way to ensure that nothing gets stolen is to stage fake break-ins in order to put the guards always on maximum alert. Of course, one has to repeat those false alarms from time to time because the level of alertness of the guards invariably decreases after some time. This method puts a lot of strain on the security guards and will tire them out quickly.
>
> The other way is to fortify the house by insuring it has strong walls, secure windows, a good fence, tight roof, and so on. These measures will be of much longer lasting effect and will not cause ulcers to the security guards.

Standard allopathic vaccination might be likened to the frequently repeated false alarms. After a while you'll have a neurotic and broken down bundle of nerves instead of a healthy security force. Maybe they'll react to the chirp of a bird and kill everything in sight (=allergies). Maybe they get so angry with you that they start vandalizing the house themselves (=auto-immune diseases, MS, Lupus, etc.)

The second option will be much better in the long run. Not only will your house last much longer (a security guard, no matter how alert, can't help with the general upkeep and maintenance of a house), it will also be much safer and resistant not only to break-ins but also to storms, floods, high winds, etc. That's what homeopathy does.

Take your pick."

No vaccine has been proven to be completely safe. Safety studies are small and only include "healthy" animals. Once the study is completed, the vaccine is given to *all* animals, regardless of their health. When you take your cat into the veterinarian, you believe the vaccines the veterinarian is going to administer are safe. Why is it that a two-pound kitten gets the same amount of injected vaccine a 15-pound adult gets? It is difficult to find a veterinarian that carries a panleukopenia-only vaccine. There is no room for personal choice or individualization in current veterinary vaccination protocol.

A word of caution

If you choose to vaccinate, keep these things in mind:

- Vaccinate your kitten once at 14+ weeks of age. If you hold off until that age, maternal antibodies should have worn off and the vaccine should be effective for life. If you are not convinced, revaccinate at one year old and you should have lifetime immunity. There is no need for annual revaccination. Vaccination of a kitten any younger is dangerous and quite possibly useless because of maternal antibody interference. Keep your kitten healthy using a raw diet, keep his environment as stress free and clean as possible and keep him away from other cats.

- Most kittens contract at least one upper respiratory infection before they reach 14 weeks of age. If so, they are quite "vaccinated" against upper respiratory viruses. There is no need to vaccinate them further. Vaccination for upper respiratory infection does not keep your cat from catching an upper respiratory infection, it may lessen the severity, but it does not prevent the virus.

- If you feel you must vaccinate your kitten, try to find a veterinarian that carries the panleukopenia-only vaccine for cats. Panleukopenia is feline distemper, a disease that can be fatal to kittens. There are several brands available of panleukopenia-only vaccine.

- The protocol recommended by the American Association of Feline Practitioners and the Academy of Feline Medicine calls for vaccination of cats in low risk situations (which is means most house cats) every *three* years, *not* annually. When you get that reminder card in the mail, take your cat in to be examined, but do not vaccinate him. Do not let the veterinarian scare you in to it. Keep in mind the risk of your cat contracting the disease compared to the risk of a vaccine reaction.

- The feline leukemia vaccine is one of the more dangerous vaccines, is not 100 percent effective and has been known to cause feline leukemia. The risk of your indoor cat contracting feline leukemia is virtually nonexistent. It requires prolonged, direct cat-to-cat transmission. Vaccination of indoor cats for FeLV is not necessary and potentially dangerous for your cat. The FeLV vaccine has been known to cause fibrosarcomas (a malignant cancer) in cats.

- The efficacy of FIP vaccine is questionable and it has been shown to accelerate signs of FIP in cats already exposed to coronavirus. Since cats are routinely exposed to coronavirus, I would not advise use of this vaccine for any cat.

- *Do not* vaccinate your cat if he is sick with anything. If your cat has been diagnosed with FUS, IBD or has an upper respiratory infection, no matter how mild, your cat is sick and should not be vaccinated. I have heard of instances where a caregiver brings a cat into a veterinarian's office for some ailment and the veterinarian suggests updating the cat's vaccines "while they are there." All vaccine vials state, *"only vaccinate healthy animals."* Are there any truly healthy animals left in this World? I am inclined to say no, therefore, none of them should be vaccinated.

- *Do not* vaccinate your cat at the time of any surgery, no matter how minor. I know of instances where animals are vaccinated at the time of spay or neuter. Believe me, this can wreak such havoc on the animal that they may never recover. This happens routinely and often results in serious long-term chronic disease for the animal.

- If you have vaccinated your cat and you see any reaction, no matter how minor, get on the phone to your homeopathic veterinarian immediately. The quicker it is treated, the better. Potential signs of reaction are:

    - discomfort at the site where the vaccine was given;

- fever (normal is 100 –101.7)
- diminished appetite or activity;
- vomiting or diarrhea;
- sneezing or runny eyes;
- sore joints or lameness;
- temperament changes;
- lumps or bumps at the injection site (no matter how small); or
- any activity not normal, no matter how minor, for your cat.

- *Do not* routinely give the homeopathic remedy *Thuja* after a vaccination. While *Thuja* is one of the "vaccinosis" (a chronic disease caused by vaccination) remedies, it is only one. In my experience, *Silicea* has been more indicated for vaccinosis in cats than *Thuja*. This does not mean you should give *Silicea* after a vaccination either. If a vaccine reaction occurs, the case needs to be taken on an individual basis and then a remedy prescribed. The same caution goes for the homeopathic remedy, *Lyssin* after a rabies shot.

"If I may venture to make a prediction, it is that 50 or 100 years from now people will look back at the practice of introducing disease into people and animals for the purpose of preventing these same diseases as foolishness - a foolishness similar to that of the practice of blood-letting or the use of toxic doses of mercury in the treatment of disease."
-Richard Pitcairn, D.V.M., Ph.D.

Nosodes

The use of homeopathic nosodes in place of vaccination or to prevent disease is not homeopathy. Nosodes are made from diseased body fluids and tissue from an individual with the disease. Homeopathy *cures* disease, it does not *prevent* it. A competent immune system keeps the body from succumbing to disease. Thinking of nosodes as a safe form of homeopathic "vaccination" is dangerous.

Nosodes, like all homeopathic remedies, are so diluted that only the energy of the original substance is left. A panleukopenia nosode is introducing the energy of the disease into your cat. This could potentially cause more harm than a conventional vaccine that injects the crude substance into the cat. An energy healing modality like homeopathy or acupuncture is deeper acting than the use of crude substances like conventional vaccination.

This does not mean if the symptoms a cat is exhibiting match a nosode that it should not be given. For example, I have used the nosode, *Tuberculinum*, with great success in a couple of cats. If you are certain your cat has been exposed to panleukopenia, then administering a panleukopenia nosode *may be* advisable. The chance of your cat coming in contact with another cat with panleukopenia is slim unless you are doing rescue, volunteer at a shelter or work at a veterinarian's office. If you are concerned about panleukopenia, take your shoes off before entering your house to avoid tracking the virus in, wash up and change your clothes before handling your cats.

It makes more sense to keep your cat healthy using a raw diet and a stress-free, clean environment. Should he come in contact with a particular disease, he will have the *ability* to remain healthy.

I have nosodes in my draw of remedies, but I have never used them. I considered it in place of vaccination at one time, but administering a homeopathic remedy without the symptoms present is not homeopathy. It is the use of a homeopathic remedy in an allopathic manner. It is giving in to fear. I prefer to put my trust into the underlying good health of my cats.

> *"I'm a very old man. I've had lots of problems.*
> *Most of them never happened."*
> *-- Mark Twain*

Treat your cat with homeopathy *if he gets sick*, otherwise, just enjoy his good health and do not worry about what *might* happen. Do not look for problems, they'll find you on their own! Do not obsess about something that is in your thoughts and may never happen.

Chapter 24 – Natural Health Care Tips

Because I am a breeder living with multiple cats of various ages and reproductive states, my cats have experienced all sorts of minor ailments, most of which I have treated using natural medicine. I almost always use homeopathy, but there are some instances I use herbs or nutritional supplements. I use homeopathy instead of herbs because there is no nasty taste associated with homeopathic remedies. Having to get a bad tasting medicine down a cat's throat is never pleasant for the cat or the caregiver. Please run these suggestions by your holistic veterinarian before using them.

Upper Respiratory Infections

Most of my cats' illnesses fall under the category of upper respiratory infections. An upper respiratory infection (also known as a URI) is a cold and can be very mild or very severe. Kittens do die from upper respiratory infections, however, I believe if a kitten that is receiving proper supportive care dies from an upper respiratory infection it may be that the kitten was from weak stock and should have died. I do not believe in using heroic methods to pull kittens through illnesses. There has to be some respect for survival of the fittest. I do my best to help kittens through upper respiratory infections, but I do lose some. All breeders and shelters lose kittens to upper respiratory infections.

I am happy to see upper respiratory infections in my kittens, no matter how difficult it may be for them to get through them. I believe a kitten has to get sick in order to develop a competent immune system. Vaccinations do not develop immune systems no matter what the vaccine manufacturers tell you. Injecting several different manmade viruses into a kitten's blood stream and expecting that to be a good thing for the kitten is a mistake. Contracting a *real* virus in the *normal* manner and then recovering from this virus with minimal intervention is what develops an immune system. It is normal for young creatures, be they humans or cats, to get sick. It is all part of growing up.

The homeopath, James Tyler Kent, says in his *Lectures on Materia Medica*:

> "You will be astonished, after ten years of real homeopathic practice, that you have so few deformed babies; that they have all grown up and prospered; that their little defects and deformities have been outgrown, and that they are more beautiful than most children, because they have been kept orderly. The doctor watches and studies him, and feeds him a little medicine now and then that the mother suspects is sugar, to keep on the good side of the baby. She need not know that it is medicine, or

that anything is the matter with the baby. So he watches the development of that little one, and grows him out of all his unhealthy tendencies. The children that grow up under the care of the homeopathic physician will never have consumption, or Bright's disease; they are all turned into order, and they will die of old age, or be worn out properly by business cares; they will not rust out. It is the duty of the physician to watch the little ones. To save them from their inheritances and their downward tendencies is the great work of his life. That is worth living for."[105]

Kittens weaned on raw food and helped through their various illnesses, inherited or otherwise, using those homeopathic sugar pills *are* different. They are more beautiful than most kittens. They feel more substantial, they act differently, and they have a very special aura about them. While it is a tremendous amount of often heartbreaking work raising kittens in this manner, it does make a difference. I am very happy to see them go into homes where they are appreciated and cherished for what they are. Those homes are few and far between.

> *"What is man without beasts? If all the beasts were gone, man would die from a great loneliness of spirit. For whatever happens to the beasts, soon happens to man. All things are connected."*
> *-- Chief Seattle*

Upper respiratory infections are very common in kittens, especially those from catteries, shelters, or other multi-cat environments. The symptoms can manifest in the eyes, nose, mouth, or lungs. Sometimes a fever is involved. The most common upper respiratory infections are feline rhinotracheitis (FVR) which is a herpesvirus; and feline calicivirus (FCV). Dual infections of FVR and FCV are common. Symptoms associated with FCV include fever, frequent sneezing, conjunctivitis, inflammation of the nasal mucous membranes, and often salivation. There are many strains of FCV with the most common strain resulting in mouth ulcers. Two strains produce "limping syndrome" without any upper respiratory symptoms. There is no vaccination for the limping form of FCV and it often manifests after vaccination for the respiratory form of FCV. Feline chlamydiosis (also known as feline pneumonitis) is a relatively mild, chronic upper respiratory disease caused by the organism *Chlamydia psittaci*. Chlamydiosis accounts for about 10% to 15% of all feline upper respiratory infection cases and often occurs with another upper respiratory infection.[106]

As with human colds, cat colds should only last 7-10 days. Except for chlamydiosis, they are viral in natural and *antibiotics are of no use*, although conventional veterinarians will often prescribe antibiotics to prevent secondary bacterial infection. Cats recover and remain symptom-free so much quicker if they do not have to deal with a drug twice a day. Upper respiratory infection symptoms usually return as soon as the antibiotic is discontinued. Like human colds, feline upper respiratory infections are quite contagious and can be spread by direct and indirect contact.

A kitten with an upper respiratory infection can be very miserable. Depending upon the severity of the infection, he may refuse to eat which can be dangerous. Herpesvirus can lead to eye ulcers that can cause long-term damage.

Some kittens with upper respiratory infections act like nothing is wrong. They run, play and eat even though their eyes are running and they are sneezing all over the place. It is best to just leave these guys alone. As long as they are eating and playing and their eyes are open and not too swollen, they are doing great. Try to keep in mind that sneezing, runny eyes, and some coughing are good! Do not suppress these discharges. Be happy for all the gook your kitten is expelling, gook is good when it is coming out!

If the kitten is not eating you need to take action. If it is because he is stuffed up and cannot smell his food you will need to relieve the congestion. I "steam" my kittens by putting them into a large cat carrier that I have encased in a heavy plastic bag. On the floor of the carrier I put a thick towel that will absorb any spills. In with the kitten put a bowl or cup full of boiling water. To the water you can add herbs like goldenseal, eucalyptus or lavender. If the kitten freaks while in an enclosed carrier or is extremely active, you should probably try another method of steaming. Nebulizers use a cold steam - you want a hot steam to relieve the congestion.

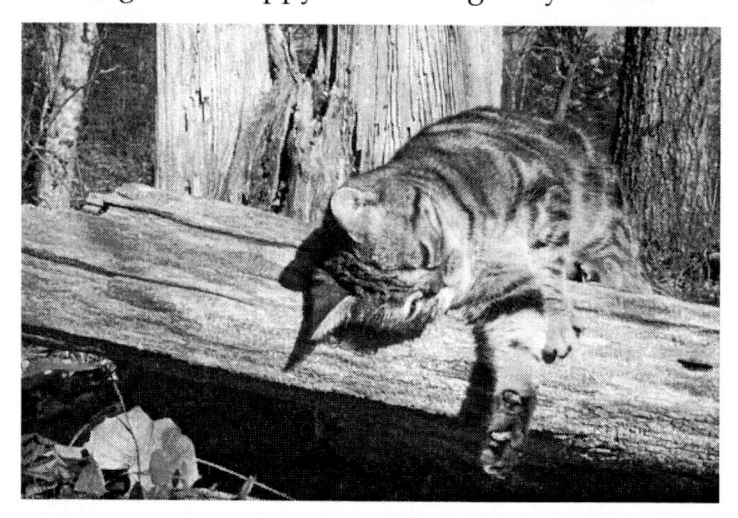

I have found most kittens settle in just fine in my homemade steam room and it is very beneficial to them. If you can steam up your bathroom without going through an entire tank of hot water, that will work as well. Steam a congested kitten as frequently as you can for about 15 minutes at a time.

You can also help congestion by bathing the kitten's nose and eyes with a homemade saline solution. Boil a cup of spring water to which you should add a pinch of sea salt and a few drops of liquid goldenseal. Once the mixture cools, sponge the eyes and nose with the solution. If you can, dribble some of it down the kitten's nose trying to get him to sneeze. Do this in conjunction with steaming.

This homemade saline solution is invaluable for any minor eye problems. Sometimes a cat gets an irritated eye and starts winking, or the eye gets slightly swollen or runny. Gently bathe the eye in the saline solution several times a day. The sea salt in the water is soothing and goldenseal has mild antibiotic properties.

Many people swear by colloidal silver as being a powerful natural antibiotic. I am not convinced of colloidal silver's powers. It should probably not be used in conjunction with homeopathic treatment. Keep in mind, an antibiotic is an antibiotic, whether it is a "natural" antibiotic or a conventional one. They are all suppressive and whatever you are using to kill germs or bacteria is not going to cure the underlying susceptibility – it will still be there when you stop the antibiotic.

If a sick kitten misses more than a meal or two you will need to force-feed him. Here are a few things you can use to force-feed:

- raw egg yolks;
- warm goat milk, raw egg yolk, and honey;
- raw liver run through the blender, warm water, raw egg yolk, and a bit of meat baby food;
- meat baby food and raw egg yolk; or
- store bought ground chicken or turkey run through a blender, warm water, raw egg yolk, and a bit of meat baby food.

All of these concoctions work quite well to tempt a sick kitten and if necessary they go through a syringe. I found a turkey baster works better than a syringe, especially with bigger kittens. Wrap the kitten in a towel if he struggles. Keep a kitten eating is important. Loss of even a half a pound of body weight is a lot for a kitten. If you are forced to feed liquid food for longer than a day or two, add a pinch of supplement powder as detailed in the recipe.

With an adult cat with an upper respiratory infection who has otherwise been healthy or is in good flesh, a fast is beneficial for them. I often do not want to eat when I have a cold. It is the same for cats. Let them fast, it allows the body to focus on getting rid of the infection.

If the kitten's eyes become swollen and red, a condition I call "raw meat eyes," you need to take immediate action. It is imperative that you keep the eyes from sticking shut (agglutinating); that is when ulcers can form. I use an artificial tears lubricating ointment that you can purchase at any drug store. A small tube is quite expensive, but cost is not an object if you are trying to avoid eye ulcers. I found the artificial tears ointment works better than the drops and is easier to apply. Be very careful when applying medicine of any kind to the eyes of a kitten with an eye ulcer. The eye is extremely fragile when it is ulcered and can rupture if punctured. Do not point any applicator straight on into a kitten's eye. Approach from the side of the kitten's head and keep the applicator tilted sideways. That way if the kitten jumps during the application, if the eye comes in contact with the applicator, it will not be to the point of the tube or eyedropper. You can also put some of the ointment on your finger and apply it to the kitten's eye with your finger (I would use a disposable plastic glove to keep it sanitary). Wrap the kitten in a towel if he struggles. I have found they usually do not fight having vitamin E or artificial tears put in their eyes because it does not hurt or feel funny.

Raw meat eyes look horrible, but as with discharges, the inflammation is a natural defense mechanism of the eye. Keep the eye very lubricated with the artificial tears ointment. You can alternate artificial tears ointment with liquid (food grade) vitamin E or vitamin A/D capsules. Just squeeze the liquid out of the capsule into the kitten's eye. If you are successful in keeping the eye from sticking it should not ulcer. If the eye does not improve in 24 hours, see your holistic veterinarian.

When the swelling goes down, if you notice a cloud in the kitten's eye, it has an ulcer. Do not panic, you can work with it. I have cured eye ulcers in kittens so successfully no one would ever know there once was damage to the eye. I have also seen and heard of many cases where kittens or cats have lost their eyes due to eye ulcers. This is not necessary! Put drops of liquid food-grade vitamin E oil in the eye several times a day for several weeks. Vitamin E does a magnificent job of healing scars. When administering anything into your kitten's eye, be very careful.

A fever is almost never a bad thing in a kitten. I am usually happy to see a fever in a cat that is sick because it means the vital force is mounting a defense. The presence of a fever will allow me to decide on what homeopathic remedy to use. If the fever goes on for more than a few days though, it will need to be addressed.

I have had very few instances of Calicivirus and mouth ulcers in my kittens. I have seen a second form of Calicivirus called "limping calici." People who vaccinate for the respiratory form of Calicivirus often see this limping form after they vaccinate. It is usually accompanied by a high fever. Since I do not vaccinate my cats against any upper respiratory virus, I expect what I'm seeing is vaccine damage from previous generations coming through the lines. This gives you an idea of how much of an impact a vaccine can bring about in the body. There is no vaccine for the limping form of Calicivirus.

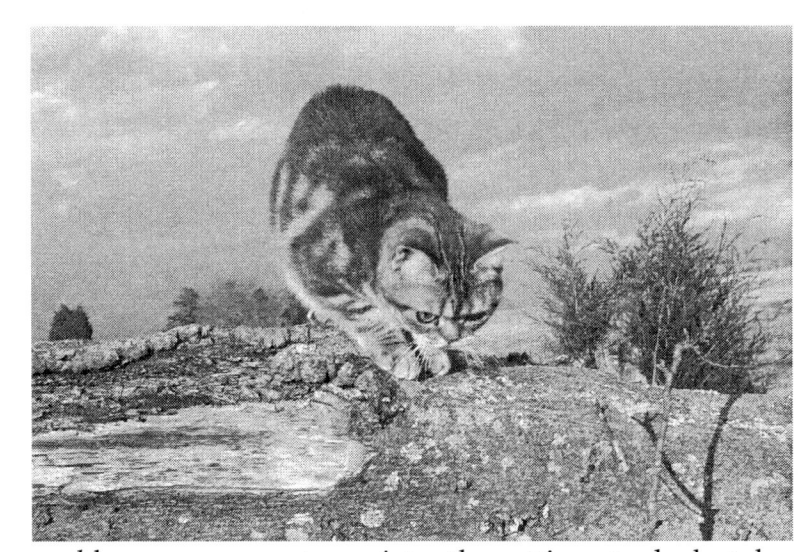

A kitten's upper respiratory infection symptoms can sometimes seem like they last forever. It gets very frustrating to see them sick. You want them better and it seems like they are never going to recover. Try to hang in there. If the kitten is eating and maintaining weight and her eyes are not consistently getting stuck shut, keep up the nursing and keep in contact with your homeopathic veterinarian. It can often take several remedies to cure a cat or kitten of an upper respiratory infection. One remedy usually does not do it. Once the acute symptoms abate when using homeopathy, the underlying miasm may show symptoms. This is the perfect time to treat any inherited disease your cat or kitten may have. Even though it seems like your cat or kitten has been sick for months and months, keep in mind that everything changes. She will get better *as long as you do not suppress the symptoms*. Natural healing takes time to work. It does not happen overnight. Your cat or kitten may be sick today, but that is not the way it will always be. Everything changes. There are no quick fixes or silver bullets, you need to wait it out and let natural healing work its magic. You will be glad you did in the end and in no time, you will forget all about the time you spent agonizing over your sick companion. In the grand scheme of things, given all the chronic disease cats suffer with today, an upper respiratory infection is not a terrible disease.

"Without accepting the fact that everything changes, we cannot find perfect composure. But unfortunately, although it is true, it is difficult for us to accept it. Because we cannot accept the truth of transience, we suffer."
-- *Shunryu Suzuki*

Ringworm

Ringworm is a skin condition common in many catteries and shelters. Ringworm is a fungus like athlete's foot and is more common in the warmer, humid climates like the southern United States. I hear of people who have spent thousands of dollars cleaning up a ringworm problem in their cattery. It does not have to be that way. Ringworm is not leprosy and you can clear it, even in a multi-cat environment, without spending a lot of money or resorting to toxic conventional medicine. I had ringworm in my cattery. I cleaned it as detailed below and I have never had a recurrence.

Kittens and adult cats that are run down, have been on a lot of antibiotics or are living in stressed conditions, are more susceptible to ringworm. If you have very healthy cats living in a stress free environment, you should never have to worry about ringworm, even if a cat comes into your environment with ringworm.

Unfortunately, humans can catch ringworm from cats and that makes dealing with a ringworm outbreak more troublesome for some caregivers. Try to keep in mind it's only a skin condition and it is only fungus. You do not need to bring out the big guns to treat it.

Like coccidia, ringworm can be spread readily in an environment that is not kept spotlessly clean. I keep a splash of bleach in all the spray bottles I use for cleaning. Bleach kills ringworm spores. Now that I am living in the southern United States and have wall-to-wall carpeting, I vacuum frequently.

Working with longhair cats with ringworm is more difficult than with shorthair cats. It is generally not a good idea to shave a cat with ringworm as it spreads the spores and can irritate the skin. Gently cut the hair back, especially in the areas where there are ringworm lesions. If you have longhair cats and ringworm has been a problem in the past, it may be beneficial to keep the cats you are not showing shaved down.

All of the cats and kittens in a house with ringworm must be bathed. There are no exceptions to the rule. I know this cure is going to put off anyone who has a lot of cats in their house or is afraid to bathe their cats. When I had the ringworm in my cattery, I had about nine adult cats and maybe six kittens. My adults never broke with ringworm lesions. The kittens looked horrible! Besides having upper respiratory infections, they were covered in ringworm lesions. My homeopathic veterinarian later confided in me that when she first saw this bunch of kittens, she did not think I was going to pull them through because they looked so bad.

I made a homemade shampoo using the following ingredients in a base of about eight ounces of lavender castile soap:

- 2 teaspoons of bleach;
- 3 drops of tea tree oil;
- 3 drops of iodine;
- 10 drops of liquid goldenseal herb; and
- 10 drops of liquid Pau d'Arco herb.

Note: you should never apply either tea tree oil or bleach directly on a cat. The above mixture contains both ingredients, but they are highly diluted. You should be careful when using any essential oil with cats, as they tend to be quite sensitive to them. Do not apply them directly on your cat.

All of the above ingredients are readily available at any health food store. Add a couple of ounces of spring water to the entire mixture and shake well.

Wash the cat using the soap and then rinse with a solution of a gallon of warm water and to which you add two ounces of potassium sulphate (see the resources chapter for sourcing information). Potassium sulphate is also referred to as Sulphurated Potash or Liver of Sulphur and is used by water gardeners to keep fungus under control. After that rinse, thoroughly rinse with clean water and dry the cat.

It is best during the treatment to keep your cat confined to a room or two. Clean every surface in your house with a solution of water and bleach. Clean every surface at least once a week for three weeks.

If you breed, you will need to stop breeding for at least six months after the outbreak. Kittens are walking time bombs. If there is any ringworm spore in the house that you have missed, a kitten will break with it.

I did not treat my adult cats with homeopathy. The kittens were all on various remedies for their symptoms. I often see the remedy *Bacillinum* recommended to treat ringworm or for use in catteries with chronic ringworm problems. This is a dangerous practice and just plain bad homeopathy. You cannot suggest to someone that they put a homeopathic remedy in a community water bowl for a bunch of cats – for any condition! It does not work that way! If you are going to treat a bunch of cats for ringworm using homeopathy, you take the case for each and every cat. Of course, that takes time and money and too many people are looking for that magic silver bullet.

As Hahnemann says in his *Organon of Medicine*,

> "But this laborious, sometimes very laborious, search for and selection of the homoeopathic remedy most suitable in every respect to each morbid

state, is an operation which, notwithstanding all the admirable books for facilitating it, still demands the study of the original sources themselves, and at the same time a great amount of circumspection and serious deliberation, which have their best rewards in the consciousness of having faithfully discharged our duty. How could his laborious, care-demanding task, by which alone the best way of curing diseases is rendered possible, please the gentlemen of the new mongrel sect, who assume the honorable name of homoeopathists, and even seem to employ medicines in form and appearance homoeopathic, but determined upon by them anyhow (*quidquid in buccam venit*), and who, when the unsuitable remedy does not immediately give relief, in place of laying the blame on their unpardonable ignorance and laxity in performing the most and important and serious of all human affairs, ascribe it to homoeopathy, which they accuse of great imperfection (if the truth be told, its imperfection consists in this, that the most suitable homoeopathic remedy for each morbid condition does not spontaneously fly into their mouths like roasted pigeons, without any trouble on their own part). They know, however, from frequent practice, how to make up for the inefficiency of the scarcely half homoeopathic remedy by the employment of allopathic means, that come much more handy to them, among which one or more dozens of leeches applied to the affected part, or little harmless venesections to the extent of eight ounces, and so forth, play an important part; and should the patient, in spite of all this, recover, they extol their venesections, leeches, etc., alleging that, had it not been for these, the patient would not have been pulled through, and they give us to understand, in no doubtful language, that these operations, derived without much exercise of genius from the pernicious routine of the old school, in reality contributed the best share towards the cure. But if the patient die under the treatment, as not unfrequently happens, they seek to console the friends by saying that they themselves were witnesses that everything conceivable had been done for the lamented deceased. Who would do this frivolous and pernicious tribe the honour to call them, after the name of the very laborious but salutary art, homoeopathic physicians? May the just recompense await them, that, when taken ill, they may be treated in the same manner!"[107]

The above treatment plan worked for me. I never had another break of ringworm and I know my cats have been since exposed to ringworm several times.

Other Minor Skin Problems

The skin is the least vital organ of the body; therefore, if you look at disease in a holistic manner, any disruption in the skin is minor. It is important if your cat has a skin problem that you keep on that level and not suppress it in any form. Most conventional treatment for skin problems is suppressive. Homeopathy or herbal preparations can be suppressive if not used correctly such as the automatic use of *Bacillinum* for ringworm.

Most minor skin problems resolve in time if the cat is on a balanced raw diet and not under constant stress. Sometimes a switch from commercial food to raw food will cause minor skin irritation due to detoxification. That is a good thing, especially if the cat had experienced a similar problem in the past. Recurrence of old skin conditions, especially when under the homeopathic treatment, is a sign of healing – do the right thing this time and do not push the symptoms back under the rug! Let them be there in all their glorious ugliness!! The skin is a wondrous organ that is constantly renewing itself. In most cases, if the cat is properly supported nutritionally and not under stress, the skin will take care of itself.

Skin conditions are ugly and if the cat is constantly itching or licking it is distracting and upsetting for the caregiver. Antihistamines and steroids do a marvelous job of making these awful symptoms go away, but it is not in the best interest of the cat to use these drugs. The problem may go away for the time being, but the chances are darn good it will come back. Antihistamines and steroids do not *cure* skin disease – they suppress it. They cover it up so no one has to look at it.

James Tyler Kent addresses the common practice of covering up skin conditions is addressed in his lecture on the homeopathic remedy *Sulphur* in his *Lectures on Materia Medica*,

> "The great mischief done by allopaths is due to the fact that they want to cover up everything that is in the economy; they act as if ashamed of everything in the human race; whereas homeopathy endeavors to reveal everything in the human race and antidote those drugs that cover up and free those diseases that are held down."

The crude form of Sulphur was once used to suppress eruptions. The homeopathic remedy, *Sulphur*, will bring the eruptions back to the surface and if the remedy was properly chosen, ultimately **cure** the patient.

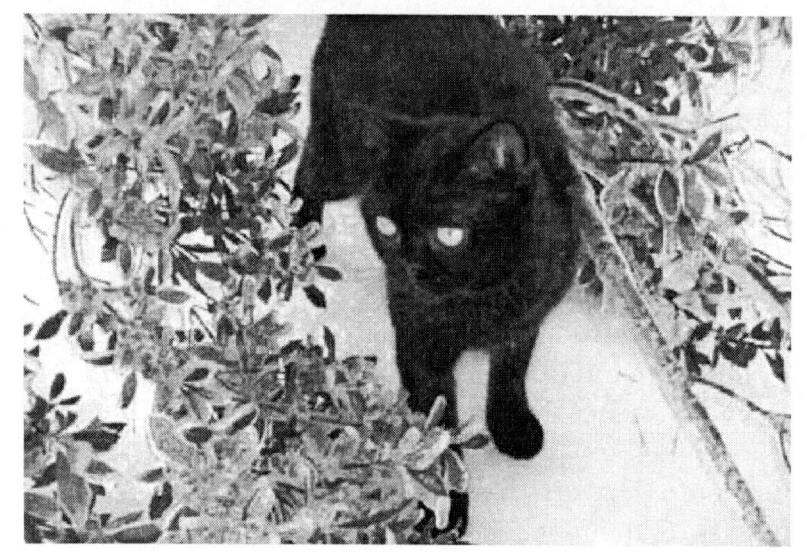

Once the cat is on a properly balanced raw diet, as long as the cat is not terribly uncomfortable, waiting out the skin problem is the best option. It usually resolves in time. You may want to keep in mind how long your cat was on commercial food. If you fed commercial food for three years, it may take as long as three months for a raw diet to improve coat quality.

Addition of flax, sunflower, safflower, or other vegetable oil to your cat's food is not going to help. Cats cannot use the omega fatty acids in plant oils. They lack the digestive flexibility to do so. As long as your cat will still eat the food (some object to a strong salmon flavor), you could temporarily add more salmon oil to the diet. The anti-inflammatory action of the omega 3 fatty acids in the salmon oil may help with any itchy skin your cat is suffering with. Be sure the meat you are using is lean and that you remove the skin and excess fat from any poultry. Chicken skin and fat is high in omega 6 fatty acids that are pro-inflammatory.

If you think stress may be related to the skin condition, double the amount of vitamin B complex in the diet. Vitamin B is extremely useful to help your cat get through stressful situations and can be helpful to skin conditions. This is not, however, a long-term fix. You will ultimately need to remove the stress from your cat's life. Stress equals illness in cats. They do not tolerate stress well. Overcrowding, lack of fresh air, inadequate exercise, disruption in the normal routine, moving to a new home, or disharmony in the human relationships in the environment can be stressful for a cat. Cats are highly spiritual creatures and are sensitive to much more than they are given credit for.

If I am stressed for any length of time, I see health problems in my cats. They are mirrors of my mental health. If I get in a tizzy over something, they get all rickety in their health. When I get my head screwed back on straight, they all get better.

The addition of extra water to the diet could help with a skin problem. An animal that is not properly hydrated will have dry, flaky skin. Be sure the water you are using is either spring or distilled water. Tap water may contain chemicals or minerals that are problematic for sensitive cats. Try putting pretty bowls of water in various places in your house to encourage your cat to drink more. If the air is dry in your house, use humidifiers.

Minor lumps and bumps are another condition that is usually best left alone. As long as the lump is not growing in an alarming manner, leave it alone. Conventional medicine likes to cut off offending pieces of the body. Lumps and bumps are common in animals that have been vaccinated on an annual basis for any length of time. Cutting off anything may be done to the constitutional detriment of the patient.[108] Lumps and bumps are very curable with homeopathy, so try homeopathy before you put your cat through surgery.

Abscesses are common in some cats and usually resolve themselves quite well by applying hot compresses as frequently and for as long as the cat will tolerate. I know the conventional treatment for abscesses is antibiotics and sometimes lancing, but cats that have abscesses treated using antibiotics seem to become more prone to abscesses in the future. It may be prudent to have the animal examined, especially if the abscess is close to an organ like the eye, to be sure there is no damage to the organ, or if the animal becomes listless during treatment signaling a more serious condition. Two remedies to consider for abscesses are *Silicea* and *Hepar sulphuris*. *Silicea* in particular has worked very well for me with abscesses. Ultimately, you want the abscess to burst and drain and *Silicea* seems to help that process along. Care should be taken when using *Hepar sulphuris* for abscesses to avoid the remedy acting in a suppressive manner. A low potency (like 30c) will promote formation of pus while a higher potency will resolve the abscess.

Fleas

When I was living in the relatively flea-free city of Boston, I thought healthy cats repelled fleas. I recently discovered this is not quite true. Fleas are common in the southern United States and now that I live in North Carolina, I have to deal with fleas. I do not resort to toxic poisons like Advantage or Frontline to repel or kill fleas. You cannot tell me that a liquid that put on your cat's skin that will in turn cause any flea that bites your cat to die is safe and nontoxic for the cat.

I use the less toxic methods of flea combing my cats on a regular basis and treating the environment with Borax or diatomaceous earth (DE). In noting the number of fleas I comb off any one cat, I can tell which cat may not be as healthy as another. My cats who are not as healthy tend to attract more fleas than others. Even though some of my cats are 100 percent naturally raised and the others have been on raw and not vaccinated (except for rabies) for as long as I have had them, I do not fool myself and think that they are completely healthy. It is going to take several generations of naturally raised cats in order to get to truly healthy cats.

Some people sprinkle DE directly on their dogs and cats. If you do that, be sure you are using a food grade DE. The horticultural grade can be used outside. Wear a mask while sprinkling DE and remove your cats from the area until the dust settles. Inhalation of DE can be very dangerous so use caution.

There is an excellent article on natural flea control written by Christie Keith on her web site **http://www.caberfeidh.com/**. Do an Internet search on "natural flea control" and you will find many articles on the topic.

Like ringworm, you do not need to resort to toxic conventional medicines to cure the problem. Although they may take longer, simple and noninvasive methods do work. Flea combing is a great way of bonding with your cat. Mine fight over who is going to get combed. No matter where he is in the house, if I am combing somebody, Rooney comes running to get combed. He does the same thing if I scratch my back using a wooden back scratcher. He has the most amazing hearing.

There are many natural solutions for flea control available both in books and on the Internet. I have tried several different herbal powders and sprays and cannot recommend any particular brand or combination. With cats, I think flea combing is the best option. You need to be careful what you use because cats tend to be particularly sensitive to essential oils and some herbs. If your cat becomes terribly infested a homeopathic work-up is in order. While a healthy cat will not necessarily repel fleas, he should not become horribly infested either.

> *"While day by day the overzealous student stores up facts for future use, He who has learned to trust nature finds need for ever fewer external directions. He will discard formula after formula, until he reaches the conclusion: Let nature take its course. By letting each thing act in accordance with its own nature, everything that needs to be done gets done."*
> *-- Lao-Tzu*

Ear Mites

Ear mites are right up there with fleas in being a nuisance factor. Luckily, my cats have remained free from mites even though they have been exposed to cats with mites on numerous occasions. There are plenty of conventional drugs available to treat mites, none of which I would use. Sometimes these drugs work, but often they do not. The ear mites go away for a while and then come back. Richard Pitcairn, DVM and Anitra Frazier recommend drowning the mites and healing the ear with a solution of oils (olive, almond and vitamin E) followed by use of a solution of dried Rue (*Ruta graveolens*), witch hazel extract and boiling water to kill the mites.[109] Unfortunately, the herb, Rue, is often used as a "cat deterrent" so I expect use of this formula is going to result in your mite-infested cat heading for the hills whenever she sees the dropper bottle in your hand.

Cats do not particularly care to have solutions poured in their ears anyway so you will probably have a fight on your hands no matter what you use. Wrap your cat in a towel if need be. Consistency is the key to eliminating mites in a natural manner.

William Pollak DVM., a homeopathic veterinarian with an office in Fairfield, Iowa recommends the following protocol:

Step 1: Make a mixture of 1/2 ounce of almond or olive oil and 400 IU vitamin E in a dropper bottle. Warm to body temperature and put about 1/2 dropper full in the ear, massaging the ear canal well for a minute or so. Let your pet shake its head and then gently clean out the opening with cotton swabs. Q-tip type applicators may compact material already in the ear canal. Apply the oil every other day for six days. Then let the ears rest for 3 days. (The oil mixture will smother many of the mites and start a healing process.)

Step 2: Using a tincture of the herb yellow dock, dilute it with water (9 drops to 1 tablespoon of water). Treat the ears with this mixture, as described above, once every 3 days for 6 weeks. Ear mite eggs are quite resistant to just about anything after they have already hardened, that is why a six-week period of treatment is recommended. The eggs will continue to hatch out in cycles and if medicine is present for six continuous weeks (medicine administered will last for four days) there will be no more eggs present.

You may need to thoroughly shampoo the head and ears (and the tip of the tail), because the mites can leave the ears; they do like to go for night trips to check out the terrain and might crawl back in after treatment. The tip of the tail may have a few mites from when it is curled near the head. Make a tea infusion of yellow dock and use it as a final rinse.

Ark Naturals has a product called Ears All Right that contains aloe vera gel, calendula, rosemary, myrrh and cinnamon leaf extracts. Annie's Herbals has an herbal ear mite oil that contains Neem and various other herbs. See the Resources Chapter for sourcing information.

As with fleas and any other parasite, the health of the animal may be compromised if he becomes infested with ear mites. Ear mites tend to be more common in kittens and should resolve easily. If your adult cat becomes infested with ear mites, you should probably contact a competent homeopathic veterinarian to address your cat's underlying health.

Trauma

Trauma includes injury from a fall or other accident or extreme fright. Cats, as graceful and athletic as they are, can still fall. Cats seem to do better in falls from very high places because they have time to right themselves before landing.

While I was living in Boston, I had a kitten who thought he could fly, fall off my second-floor back porch. Because the house was built on a high stone foundation, his fall was closer to three stories. I ran down into the backyard expecting to find him dead. He was still alive and had crawled under the porch on the first floor. I brought him upstairs, immediately administered *Arnica*, and called my homeopathic veterinarian. She advised me to watch his gums to be sure they did not lose color as that would mean internal bleeding. Lucky for me in a few hours the kitten was up and walking around. He seemed sore for a few days, but did not suffer any further consequences from his fall.

Arnica is a classic remedy for blunt trauma of any kind. The animal will be in great pain and afraid of touch. They will usually want to be alone and will be constantly shifting position as if it is painful to lie in one position for any length of time. *Arnica* is best given as soon after the injury as possible, however, it may be indicated in a chronic case if the animal was "never right" after the injury and is displaying *Arnica* symptoms.

My back porch was immediately screened in to prevent further tragedies. You should be certain your windows and porches are secure to prevent falls

I had a serious mountain bike fall many years ago. I found the biggest rock on the mountain and fell on it while traveling at a great rate of speed. As soon as I got home I took a couple of doses of *Arnica* and while I was sore, I know it was not as bad as it could have been.

Intense fright is traumatic for any cat and the remedy to reach for as soon after the fright as you can is *Aconite*. When I was showing Yukon as a kitten he had a very bad experience. While in a judging cage in the ring, the row of cages he was in got tipped over backwards onto the ground. The cages are made of metal so they made a terrible noise. Luckily, I was very close to his cage at the time and was able to run over and grab Yukon and the kitten that was in the cage next to him before they got loose in the show hall. Yukon, who was never a calm, laid back kitten, was completely freaked out (the other kitten who was an Abyssinian thought it was all a big game).

I went back to my benching cage and immediately gave him a 30c dose of *Aconite*. I carry my Washington 30c kit to shows with me. He got several 30c doses in the next hour as well as some Animal Emergency Care flower essences made by Green Hope Flower Essences (see the resources chapter for purchasing information). Although he was a bit on edge, I was able to show him for the rest of the show.

Many cats have their show careers ruined by such an incident. If their caregivers had used *Aconite* or a product such as Animal Emergency Care or Rescue Remedy, they may have recovered without long-term effects. I like the Green Hope Flower Essences for my cats because they are not preserved in alcohol like Rescue Remedy and other Bach Flower Remedies. Green Hope uses Red Shiso in a base of well water and white vinegar as a preservative. My cats will take Green Hope essences without a fight or foaming at the mouth. I keep several bottles of Animal Emergency Care on hand. I suggest you buy at least bottle to keep in case of such an emergency. Green Hope makes a whole line of animal care essences. Their New Beginnings formula is good for a move to a new home. I used both Animal Emergency Care and New Beginnings during my relocation from Massachusetts to North Carolina.

If you show or travel with your cat, you may want to keep a few emergency remedies in your show bag. I recommend at least *Aconite*, *Arnica*, *Arsenicum* (for food poisoning), a bottle of Animal Emergency Care, *Hypericum* and *Ledum*.

For food poisoning, *Arsenicum album* is helpful as is *Veratrum album*.

Bryonia should be considered for injuries where the cat does not want to move (compared to *Rhus toxicodendron* where the cat is better with movement). The cat will often lie on the injured area or will desire pressure on the injured area (compared to *Arnica* where he will not want the injury touched and may be terribly fearful of touch).

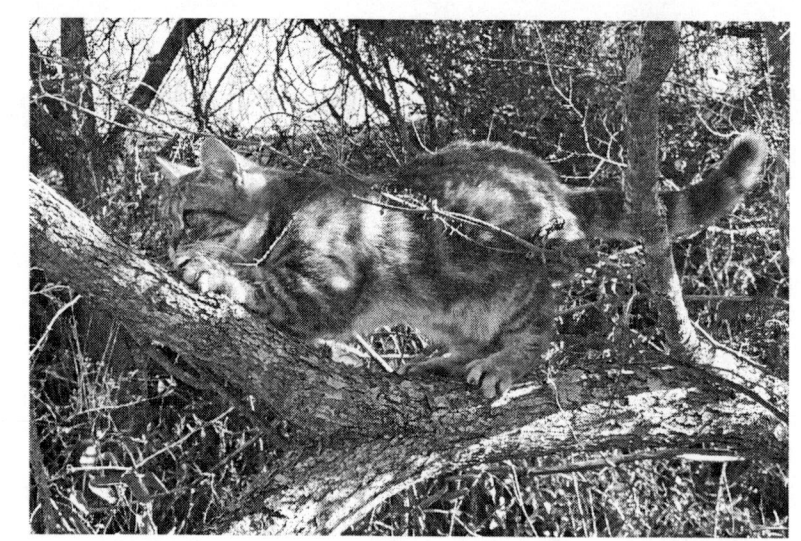

Cantharis is a good remedy for minor urinary tract irritations like cystitis. I have used *Cantharis* twice in the past for urinary tract irritations, both in females. Use caution in dealing with a urinary tract infection or disorder in a male cat because risk of blockage is serious. If several 30c doses of *Cantharis* do not work, get the cat to a veterinarian, preferably a holistic veterinarian. While I have not had success with it, *Urtica urens* is another remedy for urinary tract irritations.

For crush injuries, especially to fingers, toes, or tails, think of *Hypericum* (which is homeopathically-prepared St. John's Wort, an herb often used for depression). *Hypericum* is for injuries due to crushing or any trauma to an area that contains a lot of nerves like the teeth or spinal cord.

Ledum is a great remedy for puncture wounds of any kind including cat bites. I am allergic to cat bites and many years ago ended up in the hospital on IV antibiotics after a cat bite. Since then, I resort to *Ledum* if I get bit or seriously scratched and it has always worked like a charm.

Phosphorus is a remedy for bleeding or hemorrhaging, although in this situation, a trip to the emergency room is warranted. Nosebleeds, bright red blood in the urine or stool may indicate *Phosphorus* if the symptom picture matched.

The remedies *Rhus toxicodendron* and *Ruta graveolens* are helpful for joint pains. A cat needing *Rhus* will be better after movement. I call *Ruta* the "crushed kitten remedy" as it has been helpful in cases with kittens that got underfoot as kittens often do.

Staphysagria is helpful to help heal incision wounds such as a spay. I give a 30c dose the evening before the surgery, the morning of, and as soon after the spay as I can retrieve the cat. For conditions that "were never right since" surgery involving an incision wound or injury from a sharp instrument, *Staphysagria* may be indicated. In most cases use *Staphysagria* before and after surgery instead of *Arnica* as is more indicated for blunt trauma.

To help the healing of bone fractures and for eye injuries, think of *Symphytum*.

Vomiting, Diarrhea and Constipation

Vomiting, diarrhea and constipation should resolve by proper diet alone. Cats with inflammatory bowel disease symptoms, which include vomiting, diarrhea and constipation, usually improve dramatically when put on a diet similar to the one detailed in this book.

If you have a cat that eats quickly (gorges) and then vomits, try using larger chunks to slow him down. If that does not work, offer very small portions of food at a time and feed the cat more frequently. If that does not resolve the problem, seek competent homeopathic help.

Infrequently diarrhea, soft stools, blood or mucus in the stool, or excessive odor may be tied to the meat you are using. If you are purchasing preground meat from a company selling meat for pet food or meat ground by a butcher, that could be the problem. Cats are normally resistant to extreme illness from E.coli and salmonella, but that does not mean that if they are consuming food that contains E.coli, salmonella, or other bacteria they will not show minor signs of illness, like poor quality stools. Grain or excessive plant matter in the diet can cause soft, smelly stools. Look carefully at what is going into your cat and you may be able to resolve stool issues on your own.

I hear of so many cases of chronic diarrhea in young cats. Often they have spent months on drugs like Albon or Flagyl and they still have diarrhea! The caregivers try every type of food on the market, usually without long-term improvement. The cat is often put through thousand of dollars worth of tests like endoscopy surgery, biopsy, x-rays and blood work. They are often forced to resort to a steroid to control the diarrhea.

In young cats, the diarrhea may be due to a number of different things such as microscopic parasites like coccidia or giardia, irritation of the digestive tract from previous antibiotic use, food allergy or early inflammatory bowel disease.

Coccidia infestation is particularly common in kittens and should be self-limiting. Lack of proper hygiene in catteries or shelters can perpetuate a coccidia infestation as coccidia are spread through feces. The stool of a cat with coccidia will have a distinctive sweet smell. I can sometimes walk through the halls of a cat show and smell cats with active coccidia infections. An unhealthy animal is going to be more prone to coccidia infestation and long-term problems. I have had cats from other catteries come into my cattery with coccidia. When it happens, I get even more aggressive with litter box cleaning (bleach kills just about anything so I increase the amount of bleach in my spray bottles). Even when exposed, I have never had a coccidia infection in my resident cats. Cats that came into my cattery with coccidia were treated with homeopathy, not conventional medicine.

Kittens are often put through many rounds of antibiotics, usually due to upper respiratory infections. Upper respiratory infections are viral in nature, therefore, antibiotics are of no use, but some veterinarians will put kittens with upper respiratory infections on antibiotics to prevent secondary infection. It makes so much more sense to treat an illness if it happens instead of using antibiotics as a preventative. There was a time when Amoxicillin was the antibiotic of choice for upper respiratory infections. Amoxi is rarely prescribed these days. They go for the big guns now like Zithromax and Baytril (which can cause blindness in cats).

Upper respiratory infections need to run their course in kittens, but because today's kittens are so compromised due to generations of commercial cat food and over vaccination, they often can go months with upper respiratory infection symptoms. If a kitten with upper respiratory infection does not recover after the first round of antibiotics or other medicine, the caregiver will usually take him back to the veterinarian and a different antibiotic will be prescribed. The kitten may be put on as many as three or four different antibiotics before he ultimately recovers. I often wonder if the recovery is due to the antibiotics or the upper respiratory infection has just run its course.

Antibiotic use is detrimental to a kitten's digestive and immune system. Nonjudicial use of antibiotics is suppressive and not a good idea for the long-term health of your kitten. Should you elect to put your kitten on an antibiotic, you should be administering a high quality probiotic supplement to help counter the antibiotic's action on bacteria in the digestive tract. Use the probiotic while the kitten is on the antibiotic and for several weeks after the antibiotic is discontinued. If more veterinarians would suggest use of a probiotic with antibiotics, especially in kittens, perhaps the ensuing diarrhea that occurs in so many of these cases would not be so common.

I rarely use antibiotics and it seems almost every time I do, it comes back to bite me later on. Even I sometimes buy into the fear of horrible bacteria that is going to kill my cats and agree to use antibiotics. I cannot say there was ever a time I used an antibiotic and it helped. The symptoms may resolve while the animal is on the antibiotic, but they always came back, sometimes worst than before.

Bella is a good example of my lack of success with antibiotics. In February of 2000 she had a miscarriage and spiked a high fever. Under the guidance of my homeopathic veterinarian, I tried to get her fever down using homeopathy. I could not get her fever down so I had her admitted to a very well known animal hospital in Boston. She was x-rayed to be sure there were no kittens left in her reproductive organs. She stayed in the hospital for three days in ICU on fluids and antibiotics. Bella came home and was on antibiotics for another seven days. She seemed fine for those seven days. Not too long after she came off the antibiotics though, back came the fever and the symptoms she exhibited prior to going to the hospital.

For months Bella suffered with up and down fever and extreme lethargy. She got up to eat almost every day and continued to use the litter box. I had her at the conventional veterinarian's office many times, consulted with my homeopathic vet and tried many different remedies. There were times I thought I was going to have to put her to sleep – I did not want her to suffer. Neither conventional medicine nor homeopathy seemed to be working.

In July of 2001 I decided to have her spayed. I thought maybe she had cystic ovaries or some other internal problem and that spaying her would resolve the problem. Of course, when I took her in for her presurgery exam she had a fever. The veterinarian sent me home with antibiotics and fluids. They brought her fever down and Bella was spayed a couple of days later. Her reproductive organs were unremarkable. Still I had no cause for her illness.

I should note here that Bella was not the best of patients while at the veterinarian's office. One of her symptoms was very peculiar. Her feet hurt! They truly did, there were times I could even touch her paw pads, and she would attempt to bite me if I did. Clipping her claws became quite dangerous for me. I'd have to wrap her in a towel and put a towel up over her head to prevent her from biting me. Can you imagine what a conventional veterinarian would recommend for a cat that had sore paw pads and claws?

Spaying did not resolve Bella's symptoms. While she was on the antibiotics and fluids pre surgery she became quite perky and almost symptom free. I know why veterinarians and caregivers like antibiotics and fluids so much, you get immediate results. As soon as she came off the antibiotics and fluids though, her symptoms reappeared.

By now I had several thousands of dollars invested in Bella's health care with no resolution. As I do with all my cats when they get sick, I was studying her symptoms and running various remedies by my homeopathic veterinarian for approval. The remedy, *Petroleum*, caught my attention because of one of Bella's very strong symptoms – she got very carsick. She had extreme nausea and salivated so much she would flood her carrier with extremely noxious vomit, saliva and stool. I gave Bella a 30c dose and she improved. She had a few relapses but has since made a 110 percent recovery. People who saw her while she was sick cannot believe she is the same cat.

> *"Adopt the pace of nature, her secret is patience."*
> *-- Ralph Waldo Emerson*

I had a similar experience with Yukon and a chronic ear infection. Ear infections are extremely difficult to clear up, with conventional medicine or homeopathy. Yukon had an ear infection when he was a very young kitten. You hear the caution that you need to treat an ear infection with an antibiotic to avoid the infection migrating to the brain. A few days into the antibiotic Yukon spiked a high fever. Now if antibiotics are supposed to kill bacteria, how is it that he got a fever? I stopped the antibiotics and got Yukon through his fever using *Belladonna* and he seemed to do fine for a period of time. Yukon was having a very successful kitten career. He was high up in the Cat Fanciers Association (CFA) cat show standings. At about six months old, while I was at a show in Maine, I discovered Yukon had a horrible ear discharge and pulled him from the show. I had him entered in a show in a few weeks in Virginia. We were going to fly down there and compete against the cream of the crop of kittens. That ear infection had to go! First I tried homeopathy. It did not work (at least not as fast as I needed it to) so I took him to a conventional veterinarian on an emergency basis. The veterinarian prescribed several different drugs, both internally and topically. In no time Yukon was running from me whenever I approached to avoid the nasty tasting medicine and having his ears messed with. He even became head shy for a while.

To make a long story short, the conventional medicine did not cure the ear infection and we did not make it to the show in Virginia. Yukon did not make it to another kitten show because of this ear infection and missed out on a

Regional kitten win by a few hundred points. I went back to homeopathy and in time, his ear infection was cured and has never reappeared.

There is a place for antibiotics, but I do not think anyone can question that they are often overused in animals and humans.

Inflammatory bowel disease was once a disease of old cats, but it is now quite common in young cats. If a cat is taken off commercial food, especially commercial dry food, and put on a diet similar to the one detailed in this book, IBD symptoms are usually completely eliminated (not suppressed, eliminated). I see cases of cats with IBD who were treated with conventional medicine, Prednisone (a steroid), antibiotics, and anti-vomiting drugs, then go on to develop lymphoma or cancer. Conventional medicine cannot cure IBD; it only manages the disease by suppressing the symptoms.

Constipation is becoming as much a problem as diarrhea, even in young cats. I can understand an older cat that ha s been fed commercial food for years having constipation when put on a raw diet. The years of grain-laden commercial food producing bulky stools can cause the intestinal tract to loose tone and elasticity. There is not a lot you can do with a cat like this besides adding a bit more bulk to the raw diet in the form of pumpkin or chopped up wheat grass when needed. A properly prescribed homeopathic remedy would certainly help. Constipation, like diarrhea is quite treatable using homeopathy.

Spaying/Neutering

I advise kitten buyers to not to neuter or spay their kittens until the kitten is at least six months old or weighs six pounds.

While I understand why shelters and some breeders spay or neuter kittens at a very young age, I do not think it is in the best interest of the cat. I realize no detrimental side effects or problems have been discovered in early spay and neuter programs, but my definition of side effects is different than that of most people.

Caring for a cat in a holistic manner is not an undertaking for someone who does not want to put a good deal of time and effort into the care and upbringing of the cat. I believe the long-term results you achieve from caring for a cat in this manner far outweigh the extra time and effort involved.

See the chapter on vaccination for cautions on vaccinations and surgery.

Pregnancy and Delivery

Trust me – you do not want to breed cats. It is a lot of hard, heartbreaking work. Cats are prolific breeders and there is a reason for that, kittens are fragile. They die easily. It is not unusual for a first time queen to lose an entire litter. Nature took care of this problem – she will come back in heat again in a few weeks and deliver another litter in a few short months. A female cat (called a "Queen") can cycle almost constantly during the breeding season that can last from January to November. If she is not bred, she will keep coming into heat. A cat in heat is no fun to live with. She will scream and be absolutely obnoxious to those around her. A cat in strong heat can convince even a neutered male who has never bred before that he is a stud cat. Some female cats in heat will spray like a male. Some are worse than others, but there are times during the peak-breeding season that I want to lock my females in a dark closet and leave them there.

Male cats ("Toms") usually spray urine to mark territory. Their urine stinks whether they spray or not. They develop one track minds as soon as they figure out they are boys. If you have a great male kitten that you plan to use for breeding, enjoy him now. As soon as he matures, all he'll be interested in is the girls. You will lose your wonderful bed buddy. Some male cats can be aggressive towards other cats in the household, especially spayed or neutered cats. If they cannot breed the cat, they do not want it around. I know there are exceptions to this rule too, but it is normal behavior for a male cat to spray, have sex on his mind 24/7, and to want to drive away competition.

Pottenger noticed in his experiments that the cats on the cooked food diet behaved differently than those on raw food. The females became the aggressors while the males became docile, often unassertive and lacking a sex drive or they were perverted.[110] My cats go along with normal behavior patterns – the females are easy going until they have kittens (at which point they turn into savage protective beasts) and the males are the aggressors with no evident warped sexual behavior evident. They know their job and are very good at it.

Not that I recommend doing this, but you should be able to throw a female cat in heat out on the street and expect her to get bred almost immediately. That is the way cats are as a species, they are fertile and either in heat or raising kittens. Bast, the goddess with the woman's body and cat's head, was a renowned and beloved goddess. She was the protector of women, children, and domestic cats. Bast was the goddess of sunrise, music, dance, and pleasure as well as family, fertility, and birth.

Purebred cats today suffer many reproductive problems. They do not get pregnant, or they miscarry or reabsorb. They do not cycle or they cycle all the time. If they cycle frequently, or sometimes even if they cycle normally, they can develop an infection of the uterus called pyometra. Pyometra can be very dangerous, difficult and expensive to treat. Breeders try to get their females bred by different males or use fertility drugs and often meet with failure. In the Pottenger cat studies, the cooked food cats were rendered extinct by the third generation. They were so unhealthy they could no longer reproduce. Today's cats have the benefit of modern medicine to help them through their deficiencies, but many still do not reproduce normally. Reproductive disorders are a sign of chronic poor health. Many breeders use cats in programs that may be excellent examples of their breed, but who are unhealthy. Breeding to the standard is one thing, but if it is at the expense of the breed as a whole, the standard needs to be reconsidered.

A female cat should be able to get pregnant without difficulty, carry her kittens to term and deliver them with minimal assistance. Generally, mine do this. I have had a few problems, but nothing like what I have heard from other breeders.

My cats do get pregnant when bred and they carry their kittens to term. I have produced almost 15 litters since 1997. I have never had a kitten born dead or deformed. Like in the Pottenger cat studies, the kittens born to my raw-fed queens are all almost exactly the same weight and head structure. I have never had a runt delivered in a litter of normal-sized kittens. My queens take very good care of their kittens and always have plenty of milk. They retain close to their normal weight and their coats stay shiny, no matter how many kittens they are nursing. Since I have always fed raw food to my reproducing cats, this is attributable to either good luck or the food.

There are a couple of homeopathic remedies that you should have on hand for any delivery problems. The most common, *Caulophyllum* is indicated if the queen is experiencing ineffective contractions. A prolonged or difficult labor may require *Caulophyllum*. You will find *Caulophyllum* suggested in a number of books on homeopathy as well as web site to be given routinely during the last few weeks of pregnancy. Routine use of any homeopathic remedy is never a good idea. You may end up causing more difficulties for during the pregnancy.

In *Homeopathic Medicines for Pregnancy & Childbirth*, Richard Moskowitz tells of a patient who was given *Caulophyllum,* in a low potency, daily for the last month of her pregnancy. She gave birth unattended in the hospital corridor and bled heavily afterwards. Disciplinary action was instituted against the midwife who had prescribed the remedy.[111] The herb, red raspberry (*Rubus idaeus*), is often given to cats in their last few weeks of pregnancy to ease their labor and ensure good milk production. The herb, red raspberry, can have the same effect as *Caulophyllum*. Keep the remedy, and perhaps the herb on hand, but do not use them unless there is a problem.

I received a communication from a Persian breeder who, after reading a book on veterinary homeopathy, elected to follow the instructions in the book to give alternating low potency doses of *Caulophyllum* and *Calcarea phosphorica* during the last two weeks of gestation. Her queen had delivered and nursed her first litter without a problem. Her delivery after receiving these two remedies was long, difficult and her milk production was scanty. Since you now know how classical homeopathy is practiced, you will know that the practice of giving alternating remedies is not classical homeopathy.

One not-so-common remedy that I used twice, for a queen and her daughter, both during their first deliveries, is *Cimicifuga* (also known as *Actaea racemosa*). The mental symptoms of *Cimicifuga* are quite clear; there is bizarre and disabling fear that they cannot go through with the pregnancy, labor and delivery. The cervix remains rigidly closed and fails to dilate.[112] The symptoms of *Cimicifuga* are similar to *Caulophyllum*, but much more violent. With both of these queens, who were quite literally freaking out during delivery, I tried *Caulophyllum* without success. I remembered reading about *Cimicifuga* in Dr. Moskowitz's book and grabbed it. Soon after the remedy was administered, in each instance, the queen calmed down and the kittens were delivered without any further problems.

I highly recommend reading Dr. Moskowitz's book, *Pregnancy & Childbirth*. It has proven invaluable to me when assisting my female cats deliver their kittens. Dr. Moskowitz has used homeopathic remedies in hundreds of pregnancies. He provides a wealth of information in this book.

There is never a problem with weaning kittens on raw food. They quite literally fall into the plate of food and start eating. There is never diarrhea, vomiting, or other problems weaning. They start eating raw food as easily as they start nursing. There was a time that I ground all of the meat I fed young kittens. Then I realized that since a mother cat in the wild does not grind the mice she weans her kittens on, why should I grind the meat I feed my kittens?

A pregnant or nursing queen and young kittens need to be fed quite frequently. If you work during the day, feed them in the morning, as soon as you get home and before you go to bed. If it is not terribly hot, leave a plate of cold food out overnight where the kittens can get at it. A kitten in the wild is not going to eat on a set schedule anymore than an adult is. They will not starve to death.

Kittens weaned on raw meat have wonderful body weight! Their stools are perfectly formed like an adult's. To not have to deal with nasty kitten diarrhea is a Godsend.

I wish I could say all of the kittens born here at Blakkatz were delivered, weaned and transitioned to their new homes without ever missing a beat. They did not. Some got sick and some died. Kittens are fragile. In their natural state, if a litter of kittens got sick and died, the mother would be back in heat and bred within a few weeks of their death. I hate losing kittens. A little bit of me dies with each and every kitten.

> *"Normally, we do not like to think about death. We would rather think about life. Why reflect on death? When you start preparing for death you soon realize that you must look into your life, now, and come to face the truth of yourself. Death is like a mirror in which the true meaning of life is reflected."*
> *-- Sogyal Rinpoche*

Breeding is hard work. Nursing a litter of kittens through an upper respiratory infection takes many hours out of your day, not to mention lots of money out of your pocket. Feeding a litter of kittens in addition to the rest of your cats can bankrupt you – they eat like horses! My queens do not teach their kittens to use the litter box, I do, and they usually do not learn to use the box right away. They use corners of the room or wherever else they may be when they need to go. Kittens can disrupt the normal harmony in your house. Adult cats (especially spayed females) do not like kittens running amok. You may have an over protective female attacking any other cat in the house that looks at a kitten the wrong way. I know why many breeders keep their queens with kittens either caged or confined to one room.

If you are still thinking about breeding, perhaps you could lease a queen from a reputable breeder, raise a litter through their sale and then see if you still want to do it.

In summary, homeopathy can work quite well for any acute health problem. You should take the time to study homeopathy, not just the books for animals, learn the principles of homeopathy, read the *Organon* and the Materia Medicas. All of the classical homeopathy books are on-line at **http://www.homeoint.org/books**. You should get to know every common remedy like it was one of your friends. Sometime down the road, one of those remedies may very well come be your best friend in the world.

Chapter 25 - Conclusion

I am not a veterinarian, doctor, or scientist. I have done the legwork and examined all aspects of the diet included in this book. I have a very good understanding of feline nutrition, but I am always learning.

Recently I read a great bit of advice, "Avoid food that won't spoil if you leave it out. Food is organic and organic things are supposed to decay. If they do not, it's a good bet that they won't digest well, either. This goes for the stuff you feed your pets."[113] Commercial cat food is designed to have a long shelf life, it is not fresh, it is not wholesome and you should not feed it to your cat.

Using natural medicine to care for my cats goes hand in hand with feeding them a raw diet. It would seem sacrilegious to me to go through the effort of feeding a raw diet to my cats and then to use antibiotics for every sneeze. Feeding a commercial diet, non-judicious use of antibiotics, steroids and annual vaccination are all considered obstacles to cure when using homeopathy. It is sometimes hard enough to use homeopathy without adding obstacles.

I use homeopathy for myself, avoid conventional medicine and eat a healthy diet. I need to stay healthy so I can care for my cats in the manner to which they are accustomed.

If you approach anything with an open mind you learn more. If you think you know everything there is to know about something, you miss a lot. I spent many years thinking I knew everything there was to know about feeding a cat a raw diet. Was I wrong! I even learned while writing this book. There is nothing static about caring for a cat naturally. Like life, it should be ever changing and evolving like life is.

"In the beginner's mind there are possibilities,
in the expert's mind there are few."
-- Shunryu Suzuki

Caring for a cat in this manner is a lot of work. I will not deny this – but the benefits!! My cats are simply extraordinary. They glow with health and vitality. You can see their health in the pictures included in this book. All of the pictures in this book are of my cats. I cannot imagine ever feeding them commercial food, no matter how easy that may be. No matter what the disease du jour is, I will not be vaccinating them for anything I do not have to by law, nor do I plan on stocking my medicine chest with anything other than homeopathic remedies, flower essences and a few herbs.

It works. If my cats could talk, I'm sure they would tell you themselves.

Chapter 26 - Shopping List and Resources

Here is sourcing information for the ingredients for the diet:

I purchase most of my supplements from The Vitamin Shoppe. I have found their prices to be reasonable and they have the supplements in the potencies I need. Here's a list of the brands I use and the quantity I purchase. I have given the quantity because I go through some of the supplements quicker than others.

Vitamin Shoppe Ordering Information **http://www.vitaminshoppe.com/** or call 1-800-223-1216.

Vitamin Shoppe® B Complex 50 mg. Capsules (not gel caps)
Quantity: 1

Vitamin Shoppe® Dry E-400 400 IU
Quantity: 1

Twin Lab® Mega taurine 1,000 mg.
Quantity: 2

Yerba Prima® Psyllium Whole Husk Powder
Quantity: 2

Carlson Laboratories Salmon Oil Capsules (avoid brands that contain plant-based omega 3 fatty acids)
Quantity: 1

Livesvigor.com carries a multi-glandular product can be ordered on-line at **http://www.lifesvigor.com**
Quantity: 1

ImmoPlex Glandulars can be purchased at **http://www.nutricology.com**
Quantity: 1

You can order the kelp and dulse from Maine Coast Sea Vegetables on-line at **http://www.seaveg.com/** or you can call them at 207-565-2907. You will want to order one pound of dulse powder (or granules) and one pound of kelp powder. This company has a high quality, fresh product.

If you are closer to Florida, Leaves and Roots, on-line at **http://www.leavesandroots.com/** or call them at (407) 823-8840. Leaves and

Roots sells dulse and kelp powder. You can also buy psyllium husk powder from them in bulk.

Finally, in the middle of the country, Frontier Herb on-line at **http://www.frontierherb.com** sells both kelp powder and dulse granules as well as psyllium husk powder in bulk.

If you are using bone meal, Solid Gold manufactures it in one pound containers. You will want to order two 2-lb. containers.

The gelatin is available at any grocery store. Knox sells boxes containing about 20 packages of unflavored gelatin.

Farm fresh rabbit is available from Rocky Top Rabbits. The prices are reasonable and they do ship. You can order whole rabbits or gutted and skinned whole rabbits. Goat meat is also available. See **http://www.rockytoprabs.com** or e-mail Linda Smith at **glsmith@planetc.com** or telephone her at (423) 345-3292

Naturally raised rabbit and chicken is available from Hare Today Gone Tomorrow. See **http://www.hare-today.com/** or e-mail **murfette@earthlink.net**

Whole Food 4 Pets is located in Washington state for those people on that side of the world. See **http://www.wholefoods4pets.com/**

The Tasin TS-108 grinder can be ordered on-line at **www.sillypugs.com** and it is more expensive than what Northern Tool was selling it for. It is also sometimes available at **http://onestopjerkyshop.com**. If you have more than one or two cats, I recommend this grinder over the Maverick grinder or the one that is currently being sold by Northern Tool.

Wysong products are available on-line at **http://www.wysong.net** or by calling 1-800-748-0188.

Tuna Dash is available at **http://www.catclaws.com** or by calling 501-354-5015.

Homeopathic remedies can be purchased through Washington Homeopathy on-line at **http://www.homeopathyworks.com/** or by calling 1-800-336-1695; Homeopathy Overnight at **http://www.homeopathyovernight.com** or by calling 1-800-276-4223; Natural Health Supply, on-line at **http://a2zhomeopathy.com/** or by telephone (888) 689-1608; or Hahnemann Pharmacy on-line at **http://www.hahnemannlabs.com/** or by calling 1-888-427-6422

The Felix Scratching Post is available by calling 1-206-547-0042.

Animal Emergency Care and other Flower Essences can be purchased from Green Hope Flower Essences, on line at **http://www.greenhopeessences.com** or by calling (603) 469-3662

Potassium Sulphate can be purchased at Eco Enterprises 800-426-6937.

Ark Naturals on-line at **http://www.arknaturals.com** or by telephone (800) 926-5100.

Annie's Herbals on-line at **http://www.anniesherbals.com/index.html** or by telephone 919-542-4649.

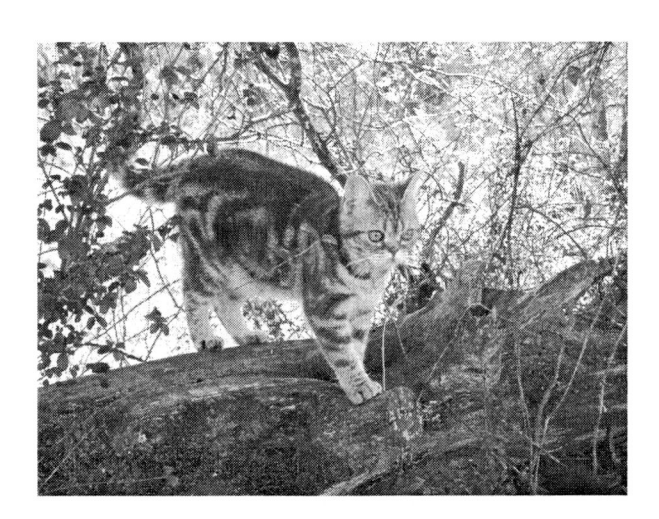

Chapter 27 – Recommended Reading

Here is an additional list of natural cat care, homeopathy, anti-vaccination and pleasure books I recommend.

To start off your natural cat book collection, I highly recommend *The New Natural Cat* by Anitra Frazier. This is *the* book on natural feline husbandry.

Your second purchase should probably be *Dr. Pitcairn's Complete Guide to Natural Health for Dogs and Cats* by Richard H. Pitcairn and Susan Hubble Pitcairn. This book has good information on homeopathic remedies for various ailments.

Homeopathic Care for Cats and Dogs: Small Doses for Small Animals written by Don Hamilton is one of the newer books on homeopathy for animals. Like Dr. Pitcairn's book, Dr. Hamilton gives remedy suggestions for various ailments. Dr. Hamilton's explanation of the disease process and vaccine dangers alone is worth the price of the book.

The information Ann Martin provides on the pet food industry in *Food Pets Die for: Shocking Facts About Pet Food* is excellent.

All You Ever Wanted to Know About Herbs for Pets, written by Mary L. Wulff-Tilford and Gregory L. Tilford is a great book. Before using herbs for your cat, please read this book.

Four Paws Five Directions: A Guide to Chinese Medicine for Cats and Dogs by Cheryl Schwartz is a good book if you are interested in Chinese Medicine for dogs and cats.

Pottenger's Cats: A Study in Nutrition details the studies conducted by Francis M. Pottenger. This book is also available via the *Price-Pottenger Foundation*, http://www.price-pottenger.org/ or by calling 1-800-366-3748.

Homeopathic First Aid for Animals by Kaetheryn Walker is a wonderful book to have on hand for emergencies.

What to learn what your cat really has to say? Read *Conversations with Cat: An Uncommon Catalog of Feline Wisdom* by Kate Solisti-Mattelon. *The Holistic Animal Handbook* co-authored by Kate Solisti-Mattelon and her husband, Patrice Mattelon, is an excellent resource for homemade food, Bache Flower Remedies and other natural health care.

Both *The Wild Life of the Domestic Cat* by Roger Tabor and *The Domestic Cat – The Biology of its Behaviour* edited by Dennis C. Turner and Patrick Bateson provide a fascinating look at the true nature of the panther sitting on your lap.

Everybody's Guide to Homeopathic Medicines: Safe and Effective Remedies for You and Your Family by Stephen Cummings and Dana Ullman is an excellent introduction to using homeopathy.

Homeopathic Medicines for Pregnancy & Childbirth is written by Richard Moskowitz. MD. This book has proven to be invaluable in assisting with birthing kittens. Remember, homeopathy works the same for cats as it does for humans. Dr. Moskowitz recently published a new book *Resonance* which is a systematic treatise on the homeopathic point of view. It covers both philosophy and method. I enjoyed the case studies Dr. Moskowitz presents in the book.

Pocket Manual of Homeopathic Materia and Repertory by William Boerick is one of the "must haves" for anyone studying homeopathy. I have had this book for years and use constantly.

J.T. Kent's *Repertory of the Homoeopathic Materia* is another book that should be on the shelf.

The *Organon of the Medical Art* by Samuel Hahnemann is the homeopathic bible. I recommend the translation by Wenda Brewster O'Reilly (Editor) and Steven R. Decker, Birdcage Books; (May 10, 2001).

Lectures on Materia Medica by James Kent is another version of materia medica for your homeopathy collection. Kent's writings offer a more personalized approach to various remedies.

While I do not own *Homeopathic Drug Pictures* by Margaret L. Tyler, the book contains excerpts and cases from books and articles by important homeopathic doctors like Hahnemann, Allen and Hering.

Science of Homeopathy by George Vithoulkas explains how homeopathy is an energy medicine and how it works. This is a challenging book and probably not for beginners. Mr. Vithoulkas wrote another book on homeopathy called *A New Model for Health and Disease* that connects the increase of various chronic diseases to the weakening of the immune system from over-prescription of powerful drugs.

A Shot in the Dark by Harris L. Coulter is a book about the dangers of the pertussis vaccine for children. Even though it is a book about the dangers of human vaccination, the same principals apply for our animals. This is a very good book to read.

I read **What Vets Don't Tell You About Vaccines** by Catherine O'Driscoll back when I was thinking maybe I should give my kittens just one vaccination. Read this book and see if you vaccinate another animal. This book was previously entitled, *Who Killed the Darling Buds of May?*

Red Cat White Cat is an illustrated children's book by Peter Mandel and Clare Mackey. I love the illustrations!!! If you can find this book, buy it. It will bring a smile to your face.

A Snowflake in My Hand by Samantha Mooney is a tear jerker. Ms. Mooney addresses "quality of life" in her treatment of animals, especially cancer patients, at New York's Animal Medical Center. This book was out of print for a while, but thankfully it has been reprinted.

All My Patients Are Under the Bed written by Louis J. Camuti, a veterinarian who did house calls in New York City. I wish Dr. Camuti could have been my vet! This is a wonderful book.

The Wild Road is a feline fantasy by Gabriel King. You will love to read about Tag's adventures. The sequel, **The Golden Cat** is every bit as good. If you like feline science fiction, check out **Tailchaser's Song** by Tad Williams.

About the Author

Michelle Bernard has spent over a decade digging into what makes cats bloom naturally with excellent health. A freelance writer who breeds and shows American Shorthairs, she has been keeping her own cats vibrantly healthy using a raw meat diet, homeopathy, and plain common sense since 1993. Michelle is renowned for her sound approach to rearing cats and her writing on many aspects of holistic cat care. Michelle offers nutritional and natural health consultations from her home in North Carolina.

Shown in the picture with Michelle are left to right, Nocturne, Moon and Wiley.

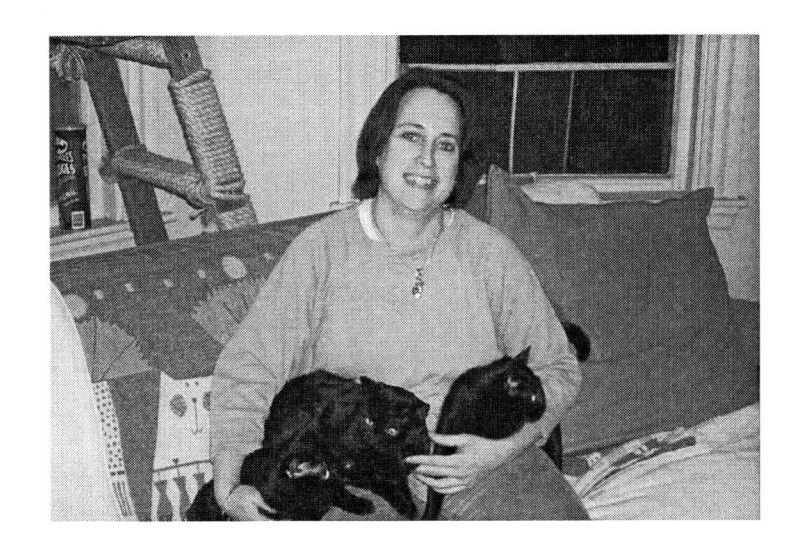

Index

AAFCO, 8, 38
Abscesses, 121
Academy of Feline Medicine, 107
acidic, 31, 49
   digestive system, 52
Aconite, 125
Actaea racemosa, 134
acupuncture, 95
acute
   disease, 91
Addiction, 72
adult food, 6
Advantage, 122
aggravation, 94
aggravations, 93, 95
aggressive, 132
AIDS, 54
alaria, 15
Albon, 127
alfalfa, 10
alfalfa pellets
   Litter, 100
alkaline, 31, 49, 53
allergies, 23, 24
aloe, 10
aloe vera gel, 124
Alpha Linolenic Acid, 39
American Association of Feline
   Practitioners, 107
Amoxicillin, 128
anchovies, 39
Animal Emergency Care, 125
Annie's Herbals, 124
antibiotic, 10, 22, 87, 113
   sulfa, 57
antibiotics, 3, 16, 24, 55, 111, 121, 136
anti-diarrhea, 87
antihistamine, 87
Antihistamines, 119
anti-inflammatory, 120
antioxidant, 29
anti-vomiting, 87
apples, 50
arachidonic acid, 7, 38

Arachidonic Acid, 39
arginine, 7, 33
Arginine, 36
Ark Naturals, 124
Arnica, 124, 126, 127
arsenic, 93
Arsenicum, 126
artificial tears lubricating ointment, 114
ASPCA, 10
Association of American Feed Control
   Officials, 8
avidin, 57
Bacillinum, 117, 119
bacteria, 29, 31, 49, 53, 87
Bacteria, 29
BARF, 94
Bast, 132
Baytril, 128
beans, 49, 50
beef, 16, 18
   heart, 19, 36
   kidney, 19
   stew, 44
beet pulp, 48
   Litter, 100
Bella, 129
Belladonna, 130
beta-carotene, 7
bile salt, 33
biotin, 57, 62
black currant oil, 39
Blakkatz, 9, 45, 135
bleach, 116, 128
blood, 18, 35
Blue green algae, 59
bone, 12
bone meal, 21, 22, 60
borage oil, 38
Borax, 122
boron, 21
brain, 13, 33, 35
breeders, 7, 17
breeding, 8
brown algae, 35

brown rice, 49
Bryonia, 126
Buddhism, 92
bumps, 121
butcher, 28, 56
Ca:P, 14
cabbage, 50
caged, 135
Calcarea phosphorica, 134
calcium, 18, 21, 60
calcium carbonate, 60
calcium citrate, 24, 60
calcium lactate, 60
calcium oxalate urolithiasis, 18
calcium supplement, 21
calcium to phosphorus ratio, 26, 31
calcium-phosphorus, 14
calendula, 124
Calicivirus, 114
cancer, 4, 54, 131
Cantharis, 126
carbohydrates, 4, 14, 46, 48
cardiac function, 33
Carefresh Pet Bedding, 100
Carlson, 59
carnassial, 46
Carnitine, 37
Carnivora, 7
carnivorous cows, 48
Cat Country
   Litter, 100
Cat Fanciers Association, 130
Cat Works
   Litter, 100
catfish, 18, 19
catteries, 111
Caulophyllum, 133, 134
Cave, Stephanie, 104
cecum, 47
cellulose, 47, 48
charcoal, 17
Cheetahs, 21
chemical, 17
chicken
   backs, 24, 26
   carcass, 21

heart, 35
liver, 35
necks, 24, 26, 31, 44
skin, 38
wings, 24, 26, 31, 44
Chicken
   gizzards, 42
chicken by-product, 6
chicken crumbles
   Litter, 100
chicken digest, 6
chicken flavor, 6
chicken liver, 13
chicken meal, 6
chicory, 10
Chinese, 35
Chinese medicine, 95
Chlamydia psittaci, 111
Chlamydiosis, 111
chronic
   disease, 91
chronic disease, 89
chronic illness, 22
Cimicifuga, 134
cinchona, 86
cinnamon leaf, 124
citrus, 50
Clay, 99
clay clumping, 99
cleaver, 27
coat
   condition, 57
coccidia, 38, 54, 128
cod liver oil, 39
Co-enzyme Q-10, 32
collagen, 21
colloidal silver, 113, 117
commercial cat food, 3, 4
confinement, 22
conjunctivitis, 111
constipated, 26, 31
constipation, 22, 24, 127
Constipation, 131
constitutional remedy, 92
contamination, 28
copper, 21, 22

corncob husks
    Litter, 100
Cornish Game Hen, 31
Cornish Game Hens, 19, 31, 44
coronavirus, 107
Cosmic Catnip
    scratching post, 103
cottage cheese, 19
couch potatoes, 89
coughing, 90
Coulter, Harris, 104
covered litter boxes, 101
cranberries, 11
crickets, 45
cycle, 132
cysteine, 33
cystic ovaries, 129
cystine, 37
dairy products, 50
Dairy products, 20
deadly nightshade, 93
deer, 12
denatured, 17
dental deformity, 24
dental diet, 6
dental disease, 4, 49
dental problems, 23
desert, 5
detoxification, 119
Devon School for Homeopathy, 95
diabetes, 4
diabetic, 51
diarrhea, 19, 22, 24, 26, 87, 127, 129, 131, 134
Diarrhea, 90
diatomaceous earth, 122
digestive organs, 29
dilated cardiomyopathy, 29
docosahexaenoic acid, 38, 59
Docosahexaenoic Acid, 39
downed cows, 17
Dry food junkies, 73
dulse, 14, 15, 21, 59
E.coli, 52, 127
ear infection, 130
ear mites, 124

Ear mites, 123
Ears All Right, 124
Ecofresh Cat Litter, 100
egg white, 57
egg yolks, 12, 13
eggs, 50
eicosapentaenoic acid, 38, 59
Eicosapentaenoic Acid, 39
Eschericia coli, 52
eucalyptus, 112
eye ulcers, 112
eyes, 13
Farmed salmon, 40
fat, 12, 38
fatty liver disease, 69, 72
FDA, 17
feed trials, 3
feline calicivirus, 111
Feline chlamydiosis, 111
Feline Future, 8, 56, 63, 65
Feline Lower Urinary Tract Disease, 49
Feline Pine, 100
feline rhinotracheitis, 111
feline urinary tract disease, 89
Feline Urological Syndrome, 49
Felix
    Scratching Post, 103
Feloidea, 7
FeLV, 107
fermented, 51
fever, 111, 114, 129
fiber, 47, 48
fibrosarcomas, 107
FIP, 107
fish, 18, 50
Flagyl, 127
flatulence, 49
flax oil, 38, 40, 120
flea deterrent, 10
fleas, 10, 122, 124
flies, 45
flower essences, 136
fluoride, 21
food grade hydrogen peroxide, 54
FOS, 51
Frazier, Anitra, 123

free range
  meat, 53
free-feeding, 9
fright, 124
Frontline, 122
fructooligosaccharides, 51
fruits, 50
FUS, 6, 107
gall bladders, 45
game animals, 12
Gamma Linolenic Acid, 39
garlic, 9, 10
gastrointestinal tracts, 23
Gelatin, 21, 61
germs, 87
giardia, 128
gingivitis, 23
glandular, 61
glucokinase, 47
gluten, 47
goat milk, 113
goldenseal, 112, 117
gorges, 127
grain, 16, 40
Grain, 127
grains, 9, 10, 46, 50, 74
grape seed extract, 54
grape seed oil, 39
grass, 13, 49
grass fed, 16, 29, 56
graze, 9
grazing animals, 12
Great Mews
  Litter, 100
Greco, Deborah S., DVM, 51
Greco, Deborah S., DVM, 4
green algae, 35
Green Hope Flower Essences, 125
growth hormones, 16
Hahnemann Pharmacy, 96
Hahnemann, Samuel, 86, 88, 90, 93, 117
hairball control, 50
hairball reduction, 8
Hamilton, Donald,, 104
heart, 33, 34, 35

heart formula, 6
hearts, 45
Heinz Body Anemia, 10
Hepar sulphuris, 121
hepatic enzymes, 7
hepatic lipid, 37
herbivores, 47
herbs, 136
herpesvirus, 111
hexokinase, 47
high fiber diet, 33
homeopathic, 136
homeopathic vaccination, 108
homeopathy, 9, 22, 24, 86, 121, 135, 136
Homeopathy Overnight, 96
honey, 113
human grade meat, 7
Hydroxyapatite, 21
hydroxyproline, 21
hyperammonemia, 36
Hypericum, 126
Iams, 6
IBD, 4, 16, 107
immune function, 33, 42
inflammation, 87
inflammatory bowel disease, 4, 36, 89, 127, 128
Inflammatory bowel disease, 131
insects, 35, 44
Insoluble fibers, 50
insulin, 4
Internet, 10
intestinal tract
  elasticity, 131
  lengthening, 22
  tone, 131
intestinal tract, elasticity, 22
intestinal transit time, 48
intra-nasal vaccines, 105
iodine, 59, 117
iron, 14, 59
Jack Mackerel, 18
Keith, Christie, 122
kelp, 14, 15, 21, 59
Kent, James Tyler, 110, 119

kidney disease, 4
kitchen shears, 30
kitten, 8, 106
kitten food, 6
kittens, 8, 134
Kittens, 56, 69, 72
Kurz, Chris, 105
laboratory, 8
laboratory animals, 93
lamb, 18, 19, 44
lancing, 121
lavender, 112
leaner, 12
Ledum, 126
lethargy, 26
leukemia, 107
Levy, Jeffrey, DVM, 9, 72
Levy, Juliette de Bairacli, 18
Like Cures Like, 86
limping calici, 114
limping syndrome, 111
linoleic acid, 7, 38
Linoleic Acid, 39
Linolenic Acid, 39
liquid method, 97, 98
litter box odor, 9
liver, 21, 41, 45
liver disfunction, 37
Liver of Sulphur, 117
L-Lysine, 32
lower urinary tract formulas, 6
lumps, 121
lymphoma, 131
lysine, 37
Lysol, 53
Lyssin, 108
mackerel, 19, 39
magnesium, 18, 21
Maine Coast Sea Vegetables, 60
malar arches, 23
malaria, 86
manganese, 21
margarine, 39
Materia Medica, 135
maternal antibodies, 106
McDonough, Patrick L., 53

Meat, 12
melanin, 37
mercury, 93
methionine, 33
Methionine, 37
Mexican, 35
miasm, 115
Miasm, 90
mice, 4, 8, 45, 134
Mice, 40
microbial fermentation, 47
microwave, 31
miscarry, 133
molars, 46
Moskowitz, Richard, 133
moths, 45
mouse, 5, 18, 34, 46, 47, 48
mouth ulcers, 114
muscle meat, 12
myrrh, 124
natural prey, 10
Nebulizers, 112
Neem, 124
nervous system, 33
neuter, 8, 131
New Beginnings, 125
niacin, 14, 33, 59, 62
nori, 15
nosodes, 108
nutritionally balanced, 6
O'Driscoll, Catherine, 104
oat bran, 50
oats, 51
obese, 37
obesity, 4
obligate carnivore, 4, 7, 8, 31
obligate carnivores, 46
obstacles to cure, 136
omega 3, 38
omega 3 fatty acids, 13
omega 6, 38
omega fatty acids, 120
onion, 10
optic nerves, 13
oral disease, 4
orbital arches, 23

organ meat, 12, 45
organic, 56
   meat, 53
Organic, 16, 42
Organon, 135
Organon of Medicine, 88, 117
ossein, 61
overcrowding, 53, 93
over-vaccination, 22
overweight cat, 69
oxalate crystals, 6
oxidation, 61
   salmon oil, 59
oxidization, 29, 30
oxidize, 28
oxidized, 29
oxygenate, 29
palatable, 72
panleukopenia, 105, 107, 109
parasite, 124
parsley, 9
Patience, 91
Pau d'Arco, 117
peanut shells, 48
pears, 50
peas, 50
Peruvian bark, 86
pet sitter, 19
Petroleum, 130
phenylalanine, 37
Phillips, Tom, 104
phosphorus, 18, 21, 60
Phosphorus, 126
pine cleaners, 53
Pitcairn, Richard, 104
Pitcairn, Richard, DVM, 10, 123
plants, 35
Pollak, William, DVM, 123
pork, 18
potassium, 14, 21, 33, 59
potassium sulphate, 117
Pottenger, Francis M., 1, 23, 24, 132
poultry by-product, 6
poultry shears, 30
predators, 49
Prednisone, 131

pregnant, 8, 9, 133, 134
   cats, 69
Pregnant, 8
prescription diet, 6, 51, 89
prescription diets, 50
prescription foods, 6
Prescription foods, 6
prey, 26
prey night, 42
probiotic, 128
pro-inflammatory, 120
protein, 12
provings, 93
psyllium, 50, 51
psyllium husk powder, 48, 50, 51, 56, 58
pumpkin, 24, 131
Pumpkin, 9, 72
pyridoxine, 62
quail, 44
queen, 134
Queen, 132
rabbit, 12, 28
rabbits, 45
rabies, 104, 122
rancid
   salmon oil, 59
rat, 47
rat carcasses, 11
raw meat eyes, 113
raw pet food, 28
reabsorb, 133
recipe, 8
red algae, 35
red raspberry, 133
Red Shiso, 125
Repertory, 93
reproduction, 33
reproductive problems, 133
Rescue Remedy, 125
retina, 13
Rhus toxicodendron, 126, 127
riboflavin, 62
ringworm, 122
Ringworm, 115
rodents, 44

Rooney, 9, 31, 45, 103, 122
root vegetables, 50
rosemary, 124
Rubus idaeus, 133
Rue, 123
runny eyes, 90
rusted, 37
Ruta graveolens, 127
safflower oil, 40, 120
saline solution, 112
salivary amylase, 46
salmon, 39
salmon oil, 31, 38, 45, 120
Salmon oil, 59
salmonella, 17, 52, 53, 127
salmonellosis, 53
sardines, 39
SCFA, 51
Scheibner, Viera, 104
Schultz, Ronald, 104
Science Diet, 6
sea salt, 112
senior, 9
sensitive formula, 6
sensitive stomach, 8
shedding, 9
shelters, 111
short chain fatty acids, 47, 51
show cats, 8
silica, 21
Silicea, 108, 121
Similia Similibus Curentur, 86
sisal rope, 103
slippery elm, 24
smelt, 18, 19
snake poisons, 93
Sneezing, 90
sodium, 21
sodium bentonite, 48
Solid Gold, 60
Soluble fiber, 50
spay, 8, 131
species-appropriate, 8, 11
spinal cord, 13
spleens, 45
spray, 132

squab, 44
squirrel, 12
St. John's Wort, 126
Staphysagria, 127
starches, 47
steam, 112
stepladder
   scratching post, 103
steroids, 24, 55, 87, 88, 90, 119, 136
stomach upset, 19
stool
   bloody, 26
   mucus, 26
   smelly, 26
stress, 93, 120
struvite crystals, 6
struvite urinary crystals, 18
succussion, 93
suffering, 92
Sulphur, 119
Sulphurated Potash, 117
sunflower oil, 120
survival of the fittest, 110
Swheatscoop, 99
Symphytum, 127
symptom picture, 87
T gondii, 54
Tangle, 46, 105
tap water, 57
tartar build-up, 23
taurine, 7, 15, 29, 30, 33, 34, 35, 42
tea tree oil, 117
telephone consultations, 95
The New Natural Cat, 9
threonine, 21
Thuja, 108
tomato, 11
tomato pomace, 48
Toms, 132
Tootsie Roll, 25
Tootsie Roll stools, 48
Toxoplasma gondii, 54
Toxoplasmosis, 54
Trauma, 124
trichinosis, 18
Trompe, 44

tryptophan, 62
Tuberculinum, 108
tuna, 39, 74
Tuna Dash, 74
turkey baster, 113
Tyrosine, 37
ulcer, 114
underlying susceptibility, 90
upper respiratory infection, 87, 106, 107, 110, 135
urea cycle, 36
urinary pH, 11, 49
urinary tract disease, 5
urinary tract disorder, 4
urinary tract infection, 102
Urtica urens, 126
vaccinate, 88
vaccinating, 136
vaccination, 131, 136
vaccine miasms, 90
vaccines, 24
vegetable oil, 40
vegetables, 9, 10, 46, 50, 74
Vegetables, 48
venison, 12
Veratrum album, 126
vital force, 91, 114
vitamin A, 7, 41, 59
vitamin A/D capsules, 114
vitamin B complex, 120
vitamin B2, 62
vitamin B3, 62
vitamin B6, 62

vitamin C, 10, 74
vitamin D, 38, 59
vitamin E, 13, 29, 30, 31, 45, 56, 114, 123
Vitamin E, 29, 61
vitamin/mineral supplement, 9
vomiting, 26, 87, 90
Vomiting, 127
Washington 30c kit, 96
weaning, 9, 134
wheat, 47
wheat bran, 50
wheat grass, 48
wild rabbit, 13
Wiley, 44, 70
Winn Feline Foundation, 28
witch hazel, 123
wood shavings, 100
wood stove pellets, 100
World's Best Cat Litter, 99
worms
    round, 52
    tape, 52
Wysong, 19
    Archetype, 73
    F-Biotic, 74
yeast, 10
Yellow Dock, 123
Yerba Prima, 56
yucca, 10
Yukon, 12, 52, 70, 125, 130
zinc, 21, 22, 42
Zithromax, 128

[1] Pottenger, Francis M., *Pottenger's Cats: A Study in Nutrition*, 2nd ed., Price-Pottenger Nutrition Foundation, Inc.: La Mesa, CA, 1995, p. 1
[2] Pottenger, 5
[3] Pottenger, 1
[4] Pottenger, 1
[5] Pottenger, 1
[6] Pottenger, 1
[7] Pottenger, 9-11
[8] Pottenger, 9-11
[9] Pottenger, 11
[10] Pottenger, 11
[11] Pottenger, 11
[12] Pottenger, 6
[13] Pottenger, 9-11
[14] Hand M., CD Thatcher, RL Remillard, P Roudebush, *Small Animal Clinical Nutrition*, 4th ed., Mark Morris Institute: Topeka, KS, 2000, p. 853
[15] Panciera D, et al. Epizootiologic patterns of diabetes mellitus in cats. J Amer Vet Med Assoc 1990;197: 1504-1508.
[16] Greco, Deborah S., DVM, Endocrinology: Addison's Disease & ACTH Testing Procedures, Lecture Notes, March 2001, Academy Veterinary Medicine, Inc.
[17] Greco
[18] Greco
[19] Greco
[20] Hand, 479
[21] Colyer F., *Periodontal disease.* In: Miles AEW, Grigson C, eds. Coyler's Variations and Diseases of the Teeth of Animals, revised ed. Cambridge, UK: Cambridge University Press, 1990; 543-550.
[22] Hand, 491
[23] Hand, 491
[24] Hand, 303
[25] Hand, 695
[26] Hand, 695
[27] Wille Baker, N. and S. Baker, *The Backyard Predator. A guide to nutrition for companion cats.* Centre for Feline Education, Salt Spring Island, B.C. Canada, 1999
[28] Levy, Jeffrey, Natural Diet for Cats: Guidelines for Optimal Nutrition, v.2.01, 1996
[29] http://www.aspca.org/site/DocServer/vettech_0801.pdf?docID=349
[30] Hand, 708
[31] Eat Wild, http://www.eatwild.com
[32] Turner, D.C., Bateson, P., eds., *The Domestic Cat: The Biology of its Behaviour*, 2nd ed., Cambridge, UK: Cambridge University Press, 2000, p. 166
[33] Personal observation
[34] Zhao Xi-he, Dietary Protein, Amino Acids and Their Relation to Health, Asia Pacific J Clin Nutr (1994), 3, 131-134
[35] Science Daily, 1999, http://www.sciencedaily.com/releases/1999/09/990921071809.htm
[36] The Thistle, Mad Cows are Comin' to Get You, http://web.mit.edu/thistle/www/v13/3/madcow.html
[37] Eat Wild, http://www.eatwild.com
[38] USDA National Nutrient Database for Standard Reference, Release 15 (August 2002)

[39] Bird, D.M. and S.K. Ho. 1976. Nutritive value of whole-animal diets for captive birds of prey. Raptor Res. 10:45-49

[40] Clum, N.J., M.P. Fitzpatrick, and E.S. Dierenfeld. 1996. Effects of diet on nutritional content of whole vertebrate prey. Zoo Biol. 15:525-537

[41] Bird, D.M. and S.K. Ho. 1976. Nutritive value of whole-animal diets for captive birds of prey. Raptor Res. 10:45-49

[42] Dierenfeld, E.S., N.J. Clum, E.V. Valdes, and S.E. Oyarzum. 1994. Nutrient composition of whole vertebrate prey: a research update. Proc. AZA Conf., Atlanta, Georgia.

[43] Hand, 74

[44] http://www.thepetcenter.com/xra/bonecomp.html

[45] Bastian, Eric, Building and Maintaining Strong Bones: A Case for Balance in Dietary Mineral Composition, http://www.trucal.info/bonehealth.doc

[46] Zwart, P., Hage, M. von-der, Schotman, A. J. H., Dorrestein, G. M., Rens, J., and der-Hage, M. 1985. Copper deficiency in cheetah (Acinonyx jubatus). *Verhandlungsbericht des Internationalen Symposiums uber die Erkrankungen der Zootiere*. 27, 253-257; 5 ref.: 253 - 257

[47] USDA National Nutrient Database for Standard Reference, Release 15 (August 2002)

[48] Bird, 10:45-49

[49] Clum, 525-537

[50] Clum, 525-537

[51] Dierenfeld,

[52] Oyarzun, S.E., K. Self, E.V. Valdes, and E.R. Chavez. 1995. An evaluation of the nutritional adequacy of the feeding program of the black-footed ferret (*Mustela nigripes*). Proc. AZA Nutrition Advisory Group. 1:104-123

[53] Pottenger, 33

[54] Pottenger, 34

[55] Pottenger, 22

[56] Pottenger, 22-25

[57] Pottenger, 25-26

[58] Glasgow, A., Cave, N., Marks, S., and Pedersen, N., Role of Diet in the Health of Feline Intestinal Tract and in Inflammatory Bowel Disease, Univ. CA, Davis, School of Veterinary Medicine

[59] Glasgow

[60] Eat Wild, http://www.eatwild.com

[61] Glasgow

[62] Turner, D.C., Bateson, P., eds., *The Domestic Cat: The Biology of its Behaviour*, 2nd ed., Cambridge, UK: Cambridge University Press, 2000, p. 166

[63] The Proven Dangers of Microwaves, NEXUS Magazine, Volume 2, #25 (April-May 1995)

[64] Stratton-Phelps M, Backus RC, Rogers QR, Fascetti AJ. Dietary rice bran decreases plasma and whole-blood taurine in cats. J Nutr 2002; 132: 1745S-7S.

[65] Hand, 301

[66] Hand, 546

[67] Hand, 294

[68] Personal observation

[69] Hand, 300

[70] Zoran, Debra L., The Carnivore Connection to Nutrition in Cats. Vet Med Today: Timely Topics in Nutrition, 2002; 11; 1561

[71] Zoran

[72] Pike, Ian H., Health Benefits from Feeding Fish Oil and Fish Meal. The Role of Long Chain Omega-3 Polyunsaturated Fatty Acids in Animal Feeding. ifoma No. 28 May 1999

[73] Freytag, T.L., Rogers, Q.R. and Morris, J.G., Adult cats tolerate excess vitamin A with minimal toxicity. Univ. CA, Davis, School of Veterinary Medicine
[74] Clum, 525-537
[75] Morris, J. G. (1999). Ineffective Vitamin D Synthesis in Cats Is Reversed by an Inhibitor of 7-Dehydrocholestrol-{Delta}7-Reductase. *J. Nutr.* 129: 903-908
[76] Morris, J. G.
[77] Hand, 297
[78] Hand, 299
[79] Vondruska JF. The effect of a rat carcass diet on the urinary pH of the cat. Companion Animal Practice 1987; 1 (August): 5-9.
[80] Clum, 525-537
[81] Hand, 298
[82] Hand, 130
[83] Hand, 299
[84] Hand, 44
[85] Clum, 525-537
[86] Hand, 708
[87] Hand, 44
[88] McDonough, Patrick L., *Salmonellosis*, College of Veterinary Medicine, Cornell University
[89] The Feline Advisory Board Information Sheets, Toxoplasmosis in Cats and Man, http://www.fabcats.org/
[90] Feline Advisory Board
[91] Feline Advisory Board
[92] Feline Advisory Board
[93] Lamb G.A., Feldman H.A.: Risk in acquiring toxoplasma antibodies; a study of 37 "normal" families. J. of the American Medical Association 206:13005-1306, 1968.
[94] Warren K.S., Dingle J.H.: A study of illness in a group of Cleveland families, XXII. Antibodies to Toxoplasma gondii in 40 families observed for ten years. New England Journal of Medicine 274:993-997, 1966.
[95] Wille
[96] Carey CJ, Morris JG, Biotin deficiency in the cat and the effect on hepatic propionyl CoA carboxylase, J Nutr 1997 Feb; 107(2): 330-4
[97] Hand, 303
[98] Hand, 303
[99] Wille
[100] Wille
[101] Ullman
[102] Hahnemann, S.
[103] Hahnemann, S.
[104] Hahnemann, S.
[105] Kent, James Tyler, *Lectures on Materia Medica*, B. Jain Publishers, Delhi, India, 1995, 381
[106] Aiello, Susan E., Ed., The Merck Veterinary Manual, 8th edition, 1998, Merck, Whitehouse Station, NJ p. 1115
[107] Hahnemann, S., *Organon of Medicine*, 6th Ed., Cooper, Blaine, Washington, 1982, p. 121-124
[108] Kent, J, *Lectures on Materia Medica*, B. Jain Publishers, Delhi, India, 1995, 226
[109] Frazier, A and Eckroate, N, *The New Natural Cat: A Complete Guide for Finicky Owners*, Dutton, New York, 1990, p. 311-314
[110] Pottenger, 11
[111] Moskowitz, R, *Homeopathic Medicines for Pregnancy & Childbirth*, North Atlantic Books, Berkeley, California, 1992

[112] Moskowitz

[113] Lefebvre, P, *Diet for a Small Pleasure. Refusal of joy is the unhealthiest habit*, Clamor (Nov./Dec. 2001)